Praise for "Sleep to Win!"

Every once in awhile a book comes along that smacks you upside the head because it shares commonsense advice that is unfortunately not common practice. *Sleep to Win!* is that kind of book. Read it and practice what Jim Maas, Haley Davis and their colleagues tell you about getting quality sleep. It will help you become a winner—accomplishing your goals—whether you are an athlete, a coach, a businessperson, a parent, or just someone who wants to make a difference in the world.

—Ken Blanchard, Co-author *The One Minute Manager* and *Leading at a Higher Level*

In this powerfully informative book, the authors, Ivy League sleep educators, advise a professional hockey player on the importance of proper rest. Every athlete --indeed all of us-- will benefit from the detailed explanation of the ways to sleep better to improve performance. Happily, I did and surely you will.

—Fay Vincent, former Commissioner of Major League Baseball, Chairman of Columbia Pictures and Vice Chairman of Coca- Cola.

I believe your book will be a huge success and I will introduce it throughout our organization, players and management alike. In professional hockey the challenge is to gain an advantage both on and off the ice. Over the years we have developed a better understanding in the science of nutrition, conditioning and rehabilitation. Dr. Maas and Haley Davis now bring to sports the science of sleep. They share their expertise in a captivating and reader friendly manner. This is a must read for anyone who is looking for an added advantage over their competitors by understanding the value of REM and how to achieve it.

—Jimmy McCrossin, Head Athletic Trainer, NHL Philadelphia Flyers

Awesome unique look at sleep as it pertains to athletics. It's a must read for any serious athlete trying to reach their genetic potential. I, for one, will incorporate this information into my training program. The book is valuable not only for athletes but coaches and management.

—Pete Friesen, Head Athletic Trainer/Strength Coach NHL Carolina Hurricanes/Adjunct Professor Duke University

"Sleep To Win!" The title says it all! So much is misunderstood about this critical component of athletic performance. Dr. Maas and Haley Davis provide a very entertaining parable, presenting a very realistic story for all of us who work and those who play in the NHL. The research and data on sleep and its effects on the human body are presented in an enjoyable and understandable storyline which follows an NHL player thru his trials and tribulations of an NHL season, but this story could represent any athlete at any level. Any athlete that is looking for a competitive advantage needs to read "Sleep To Win!". This book provides practical and immediate applications on how to improve your game and your quality of life.

"Sleep To Win!" Is for all athletes, coaches and parents who are seeking to find that competitive advantage.

—Ray Barile, Head Athletic Trainer, NHL St. Louis Blues

After listening to you for so many years I forget how the culture of our success is due to you, from the timing of our team meals to making sure we don't nap beyond three hours before games etc. You have been a big part of our success. I have followed this with our kids and it is amazing how they value their sleep. The ZEO really showed our kids how they thought they were getting 8 but were really only getting 7. This book is a must for not only coaches but parents as well.

—Mike Schafer, Head Coach Cornell University Men's Hockey

When in competition or heavy training, sleep is the most important factor in achieving my optimal athletic performance. I need at least 8 hours of sleep a night for me to feel fully recovered and energized to play my absolute best. If I don't meet my sleep requirement, my legs feel heavy, my reaction time is slower and my ability to think and act quickly is negatively affected.

—Rebecca Johnston, 2010 Olympics Hockey
Gold Medalist for Team Canada

As an NHL player who has been through it, the book is bang on in terms of accuracy. I think it would be helpful to any athlete who faces playing a lot of games with a very rigorous travel schedule.

—Byron Bitz, NHL Boston Bruins and NHL Vancouver Canucks

Dr. Jim Maas and Haley Davis extend a critically important message: When will our society begin to truly value the health and performance benefits of proper sleep-to the same degree that we value proper nutrition and exercise? You'll read about the science of sleep in an easy-to-read parable form-a parable that is representative of so many student-athletes and professional athletes. This book is for athletes, in particular, that are known to search for that "magic bullet," consuming the latest science on strength and conditioning, nutrition, biomechanics, and equipment and technological advances. A magic bullet has been here all along-proper sleep! Put aside the idea of "no pain, no gain" for a moment. It's fun, it's easy, and it works! If you don't believe it-try it!

—Dr. Mary DePalma, Sports Psychologist, Professor, Ithaca College

Sleep *to* Win!

Secrets to Unlocking your Athletic Excellence in Every Sport

Dr. James B. Maas
Haley A. Davis

with Rebecca Robbins, Wendy Sterling, Hayley Hughes *and* Maura Greenwood

authorHOUSE®

AuthorHouse™
1663 Liberty Drive
Bloomington, IN 47403
www.authorhouse.com
Phone: 1-800-839-8640

Published by AuthorHouse   12/29/2015

ISBN: 978-1-4817-0723-7 (sc)
ISBN: 978-1-4817-0724-4 (hc)
ISBN: 978-1-4817-0725-1 (e)

Library of Congress Control Number: 2013900710

Print information available on the last page.

Before making any changes in prescribed health-care regimens, make sure you consult a licensed physician. While this book provides information on sleep strategies and disorders, it is not intended to be a substitute for appropriate medical diagnosis or treatment. If you are having a persistent problem, consult your physician and/or one of the accredited sleep disorders centers listed on the internet at www.sleepcenters.org.

To Nancy, Dan, Justin and Lauren Bastian Maas, Janet Maas Robinson, and Maryanne and Brittany Davis, whose love, support, patience and encouragement continue to make possible our journey towards enriching lives through sleep education.

J.B.M.   H.A.D.

Acknowledgments

"Sleep to Win!" is based on empirical investigations of many dedicated sleep researchers. In the past decade, these scientists have expanded their explorations well beyond the symptoms, causes and treatments of sleep disorders. Medical researchers and psychologists have started to focus on how sleep deprivation affects performance in education, at work and at play.

We have written books and articles on sleep for children and adults and worked with schools, colleges, Fortune 100 companies and medical societies to spread the gospel on the importance of sleep. Of great interest to us has been to learn how sleep education can make a huge difference in athletic performance across all skill levels, ages, and different sports. Our work with individual athletes and entire teams has been one of the most rewarding endeavors we have undertaken. It was interacting with college teams, Olympic athletes and those involved in professional athletics that made us realize we had something of value to share with people wanting to improve their skill levels, for pure enjoyment, personal development, or even to "go for the gold."

The expanding community of professionals who study sleep openly share their discoveries, working to solve the mysteries of the night and how they affect daytime behavior and performance. The sleep advice in our book is based on the shared insights of many investigators whose primary motivation is not self-aggrandizement, but rather the betterment of human experience. If this book is helpful to you, it is due to the largess and collective wisdom of our entire sleep profession. We have attempted to deliver helpful information in an easily comprehended format that should be fun to read. Those wishing to gain a deeper understanding of the research behind our advice can do so by turning to references at the end of our parable.

There are individuals, our colleagues, to whom we are profoundly indebted. Without their experience, wisdom and hard work, this book could not have been written. For decades, Dr. William C. Dement, the Lowell W. and Josephine Q. Berry Professor of Psychiatry at Stanford University, has led hundreds of scientists, like sleep and performance coach Cheri Mah, to pursue careers in sleep research. He has been a great mentor to all of us. His interest in athletics spurred us to study the relationship between sleep and performance in that arena. Another wonderful mentor, Dr. Helene Porte of Cornell University, has provided invaluable guidance to us on the physiology of sleep. And Dr. Craig N. Boss, Director of the Charlevoix Area Hospital Sleep Center in Michigan has been of invaluable help for his leadership and encouragement.

The authors wish to thank Rebecca S. Robbins for her co-authorship of "Sleep for Success!" and willingness to share background research and writing from that book.

We are deeply grateful to Wendy Sterling, MS, RD, CSSD, CDN, for her incredible knowledge of nutrition as it pertains to athletic performance. Wendy wrote the detailed and highly informative "Eat to Sleep" email in chapter 9. Her work with the New York Jets enabled us to train that team with seminars on sleep. And we wish to acknowledge the editorial researching skills of Rachel Eklund, a teaching assistant who has been involved in several of our endeavors to communicate sleep research to the general public.

Hayley Hughes contributed the basic foundation for the chapter on drugs and Maura Greenwood provided information on sleep medicine. Rebecca, Hayley and Maura are all talented athletes and were former undergraduate teaching assistants for Prof. Maas' 1,900 student Introductory Psychology course at Cornell University. They are pursuing graduate studies related in some significant way to sleep. Anna Grosshans and Ciara McAfee, also undergraduate teaching assistants at Cornell, contributed to chapters on advice for timing of practice sessions and handling jet fatigue. And thanks to Alessandra Shuster, Laura Danforth and Liz Zorn of Cornell, Samantha Platt of Duke University and Kitty Kristinsdottir of the University of Akron for their review of the manuscript and extremely helpful suggestions. Janet Maas Robinson led our team of proofreaders and provided invaluable assistance with her profound knowledge of proper grammar and style. Lisa Proper of Cornell University brought her skills to our production team for the second time on our writing books about the importance of sleep.

It has been tremendously rewarding to work with Amber Way, an unbelievably motivated, outstanding high school athlete from Charlevoix, Michigan. We were fortunate to introduce Amber before her freshman year of high school to the benefits of sleep for athletes. By the end of her freshman year, Amber managed to break four school cross country records and become one of the top runners in the state of Michigan. She attributes her success to using our advice on getting 9.25 hours of sleep and establishing a regular sleep-wake schedule. It is her actual case history that permeates the chapter on teenage athletes in our parable. And thanks to Coach Mary Plude who brought Amber and her teammates to our sleep presentation, encouraging them to follow our guidelines for better sleep strategies.

We are grateful to have the encouragement, wisdom and experiences afforded to us by so many outstanding athletes, coaches, athletic trainers and professors of sports psychology courses. Special thanks to Olympic Gold Medalists Sarah Hughes and Rebecca Johnston, Head Coach Peter Laviolette and Danny Briere of the NHL Philadelphia Flyers, Colin Greening of the NHL Ottawa Senators, Head Coach Rex Ryan, Mark Sanchez and Tim Tebow of the NFL New York Jets, Jameer Nelson of the NBA Orlando Magic, Coaches Mike Schafer (Men's Hockey), Doug Derraugh and Danielle Bilodeau (Women's Hockey), Matt Baughan (Golf), Steve Donahue (Men's Basketball), Rob Koll (Wrestling), Jenny Graap and Suzie Friedrich (Women's Lacrosse), Nathan Taylor, Rich Bowman, Artie Smith and Lou Duesing (Track and Cross Country), and Dick Blood (Women's Softball) of Cornell University, Head Football Coach David Cutcliffe and Defensive Coordinator Jim Knowles of Duke University, Head Athletic Trainers Jim McCrossin of the Philadelphia Flyers, Peter Friesen of the Carolina Hurricanes, Ray Barile of the St. Louis Blues, and Bernie DePalma of Cornell University, Athletic Director Andy Noel of Cornell University, and sports psychologist Dr. Mary DePalma of Ithaca College.

Dr. Ken Blanchard, educator, speaker, business consultant and spiritual leader is the co-author of the business best-seller, **One Minute Manager.** A close personal friend for over 40 years, Ken took us to lunch and suggested that we write **Sleep to Win!** in the form of an educational parable. It was the most valuable lunch we ever had. Thanks, Ken!

We wish to thank David G. Myers, a distinguished professor of psychology at Hope College and prolific author of psychology textbooks and articles. He has served as an evangelist and role model, giving psychology away so that others may enjoy, and benefit from, the discoveries arising from our academic discipline. Sharing our interest in sports and human performance, David inspired us to conceive this book.

We are grateful for the editorial assistance of our dear friend and colleague, Joe Kita. Joe is an accomplished author, motivational speaker, and contributing writer for Men's Health and many other national magazines. As a consultant (www.josephkita.com), Joe's constructive criticism, creative voice, professionalism, sense of humor, and ability to explain complex scientific concepts in readily accessible language were invaluable in helping us write *Sleep to Win!*

Table of Contents

Introduction

The story you're about to read is fiction. Certain names and scenarios have been changed to protect the chronically sleep-deprived. So there's no Mike Greenza who plays in the NHL, nor is there a Coach Harkwell. But as for me, Jim Maas, along with my co-author Haley Davis and the experts we'll introduce and the research and advice we'll share, that's all very real. As a sleep researcher for the past 44 years and former chair of Cornell University's psychology department, I've met (and worked with) numerous athletes and coaches like Greenza and Harkwell. So in that respect, their characters are composites. They're also representative. Despite significant research showing the performance-enhancing effects of better sleep habits, athletes and coaches at every level continue to ignore it. They'll spend thousands of dollars on the latest equipment, swallow the hype surrounding various "magic" supplements, and continually experiment with new training methods, but they somehow persist in overlooking the most basic yet effective performance enhancer of all, and that is simply getting the right amount and type of sleep.

That's what this little parable communicates.

Think of it as a new type of bedtime story.

James B. Maas, Ph.D.
January 1, 2013
Fort Worth, TX

1

A Frustrated Athlete

My name is Mike Greenza. I'm a professional hockey player–No. 19 with the Philadelphia Flyers. I've been in the league for two years now and am living my dream. Or at least I thought so until I went to my folks' house in Alberta for the holidays and my kid sister, Britt, asked why I seemed so down.

"All my friends want to come over when my big, hockey-star brother's in town," she said, "but they've been asking me why you aren't as friendly as you used to be. Are you okay?"

I tried covering up my surprise by telling her I was just preoccupied. In the NHL, you always need to be getting better, skating faster and scoring more. It's a lot of pressure, and it keeps you on edge. But deep down I knew it was more than that. Truth be told, I was exhausted–from the training, from the traveling, from everything. I just hadn't realized it was showing.

"Sorry Britt. I've actually been having a lot of trouble sleeping lately. I toss and turn, and when I finally do fall asleep, before I know it, my alarm is going off and it's time for practice. If I could only get some decent rest, maybe I'd feel and even play better."

Then my kid sister made a brilliant suggestion, something that would ultimately change my career and my life. Why I hadn't thought of it myself proved just how tired I was.

"Remember that psychology professor you had in college—the sleep expert?" she said. "You should email him."

Professor Myers...Mong...Maas! That was his name. I had forgotten about him. He'd been one of my college hockey team's advisors. He spoke to us a few times about "sleeping smarter."

You know, that's a really good idea....

To: jbm@powersleep.org
From: mGreenza@nhl.org
RE: Need some advice

Dear Professor Maas,

Hope you're doing well. It's Mike Greenza. If you recall, I took a few of your classes and also played hockey for the varsity hockey team about five years ago. Both experiences served me very well, and I'm currently playing for the Flyers in the NHL.

I'm writing because I need some advice. Lately, I've been having trouble sleeping. And the more I worry about it, the less rest I seem to get. It's gotten to the point where I'm concerned it may not only be affecting my health but also my performance on the ice. I remember your work with the team, and I was hoping you'd be willing to meet with me and talk some more about this. We'll be playing in Buffalo in two weeks, and I could leave some tickets for you–primo seats right behind the bench. It'll be just like old times! Let me know if you can make it.

All the best,
Mike Greenza, #19

To: mGreenza@nhl.org
From: jbm@powersleep.org
RE: Need some advice

Dear Mike,

Are you kidding? Seats behind the bench for a Flyers-Sabres' game? I'm there! But seriously, it's great to hear from you, and I'm willing to help in any way I can. I've been following your career in the sports pages and on your team's website. Seems like you started with a bang but have had some ups and downs recently. Since you graduated there's been so much new research about sleep and its relation to athletic performance. And if you're like most of my former students, you've probably forgotten what I taught you, so you're due for a refresher!

Send me the particulars about the game in Buffalo and when you'd like to meet, and I'll take it from there. But before we get together, do me a favor and answer the following questionnaires then email them back to me. They'll help me understand the challenges you're facing so I can better advise you. Looking forward to seeing you again!

With warmest regards,

Your "olde prof,"
Jim

The Maas Robbins Alertness
Questionnaire (MRAQ)
©2010 Dr. James B. Maas and Rebecca S. Robbins

Please indicate true or false for the following statements:

True	False	
T	F	1. I often need an alarm clock in order to wake up at the appropriate time.
T	F	2. It's often a struggle for me to get out of bed in the morning.
T	F	3. Weekday mornings I often hit the snooze bar several times.
T	F	4. I often feel tired and stressed out during the week.
T	F	5. I often feel moody and irritable, and little things upset me.
T	F	6. I often have trouble concentrating and remembering.
T	F	7. I often feel slow with critical thinking, problem solving, and being creative.
T	F	8. I need caffeine to get going in the morning or make it through the afternoon.
T	F	9. I often wake up craving junk food, sugars, and carbohydrates.
T	F	10. I often fall asleep watching TV.
T	F	11. I often fall asleep in boring meetings or lectures or in warm rooms.
T	F	12. I often fall asleep after heavy meals or after a low dose of alcohol.
T	F	13. I often fall asleep while relaxing after dinner.
T	F	14. I often fall asleep within five minutes of getting into bed.
T	F	15. I often feel drowsy while driving.
T	F	16. I often sleep extra hours on the weekends.
T	F	17. I often need a nap to get through the day.
T	F	18. I have dark circles around my eyes.
T	F	19. I fall asleep easily when watching a movie.
T	F	20. I rely on energy drinks or over-the-counter medications to keep me awake.

Results:
If you answered "True" to **four or more** of these statements, consider yourself seriously sleep-deprived.

Epworth Sleepiness Scale
(Designed by Dr. Murray Johns of Australia)
©M.W. Johns 1990–1997

Use the "Doze Scale" to respond to each situation.
0 = no chance of dozing
1 = slight chance of dozing
2 = moderate chance of dozing
3 = high chance of dozing

Situation	**Chance of Dozing**
Sitting and reading	_____
Watching TV	_____
Sitting inactive in a public place (theater/meeting)	_____
As a passenger in a car for an hour without break	_____
Lying down to rest in the afternoon when circumstances permit	_____
Sitting and talking to someone	_____
Sitting quietly after a lunch without alcohol	_____
In a car, while stopped for a few minutes in traffic	_____
MY Sleepy Score (Total Points)	_____

Results:
If you scored…
Less than 8: Congratulations! You're getting adequate rest.
Between 8 and 11: You have mild sleepiness.
Between 12 and 15: You're moderately sleepy and must reevaluate your habits.
Between 16 and 24: You're seriously sleep-deprived.

Winning the Game of Sleep

A three-hour drive from Ithaca, New York, where my office is located, to Buffalo is not usually something I'd look forward to in mid-January. But I have to admit the chance to see Mike play in person and also help him improve his game had my adrenaline pumping. We had agreed to meet for a late lunch at the Hyatt, where his team was staying.

"Mike, it's wonderful to see you! You look even bigger and stronger than when you graduated."

"That's the difference between college and professional hockey," said Mike, smiling and extending a beefy hand outside the lobby restaurant. "Lots of time in the weight room, especially during the off-season. I swear their goal is to make us into freight trains on skates."

We spent a few minutes catching up after being seated and

ordering, but since I knew his time was limited I got right to it.

"Look Mike, I've reviewed your responses to the sleep quizzes. I think you can definitely benefit from some of the new research I mentioned. But before I get into specifics, can you tell me more about what your sleep schedule is like right now?"

He laughed and rolled his eyes. "Well, with morning practices, night games, weekend day games, and all the travel – one night we'll be in New York and the next we'll be in Los Angeles – maintaining a regular sleep schedule is just about impossible. And I didn't even mention the charity events, media interviews, and my girlfriend who's in Toronto. I spend a lot of time with her when I'm there. Even when I do manage to get to bed at a reasonable hour, I often have trouble falling asleep or I wake up in the middle of the night thinking about what happened in the game or what I have to do tomorrow...."

He shrugged his massive shoulders. Despite his size, he did look tired. I could see it in his eyes.

"Let me give you a brief refresher on what I call my 'Golden Rules of Sleeping Well,'" I said. "It's critically important that you take sleep seriously and make it a priority. Believe it or not, sleep is essential to peak athletic performance.

"At your age, you're probably not concerned about longevity

or serious illness, but let me remind you that even a modest lack of sleep can lead to a higher risk of hypertension, heart attack, stroke, Type II diabetes, weight gain, and even cancer. And as you mentioned in your email, it can also produce irritability, anxiety, depression and, when it comes to playing hockey, slower reaction time, loss of motor skills and coordination, and a reduced ability to think, remember, make critical decisions, and avoid risky behavior."

"Whoa," is all he said. But that was good. I had his attention.

"First Golden Rule is you have to determine your PSQ or Personal Sleep Quotient and meet it every night. From puberty to about 26, people need 9¼ hours of sleep each night to be fully alert and energetic. Since you're a little older, you can probably do okay with 7½ or 8½ hours per night. But that's as low as you can go. Anything less is likely to affect your performance."

Our food had arrived – two large chicken breasts for Mike and a hamburger for me. He was shaking his head.

"Professor, I'm lucky if I get six hours a night. I just don't have that kind of time."

"Mike, it's a matter of valuing sleep. It's your choice, but if you add even one hour I guarantee you'll see a significant increase in your performance. Many people think they're doing fine on six hours of sleep, but when they do what I'm suggesting, they become entirely different people. Plus, that extra hour of sleep will make you more efficient, effective and put you in a better mood, so you'll get everything done with time to spare."

"Okay, I hear you," he said, "but it's not all under my control. Coach Harkwell usually calls early-morning practices, even after night games."

"That's a problem," I admitted. "We've been trying to educate coaches in all different sports, but they're pretty skeptical. But listen to this: In every case where we've convinced a coach to cut out early-morning practices, the team's performance has improved dramatically. We now know that something happens in your brain after six or seven hours of continuous sleep that improves motor-skill performance. There are these things called sleep spindles that enhance muscle memory. So if a coach schedules practices that shorten sleep, there's no way the team will improve. In fact, early-morning practices are far worse than not practicing at all. It's best to delay practicing until at least 10 or 11 a.m."

"So let me get this right," he said with a point of his fork. "You're saying sleeping later will boost performance more than an early practice?"

"That's correct. And my second Golden Rule, keeping a regular sleep schedule, is just as important as getting enough sleep. You've got to go to bed and get up at the same time every day. This will cure your insomnia by synchronizing the hours you spend in bed with the sleepy phase of your biological clock. That'll be difficult to do when you're traveling cross-country, but we can talk about overcoming jet lag a little later."

"And one more thing. The third Golden Rule is that it's best to get one long block of continuous sleep rather than a few hours here and there. It's critical not only for eliminating fatigue but also consolidating memory and enhancing athletic performance. An occasional late night won't cause too much damage, but reducing your sleep by just one hour for seven consecutive nights has the same effect as pulling one all-nighter. Sleep debt doesn't dissipate by itself over time. Just like credit card debt, it's cumulative. So if you lose several hours of sleep over a few nights, you'll become increasingly more fatigued even if you resume your normal sleep schedule."

Mike pushed his empty plate away and leaned back in his chair. "If I really commit to following these three rules, how soon can I expect to see improvements?"

"One week," I replied without hesitation. "You'll start to feel stronger, more alert, and that should have a significant impact on your game. And to make it easier, I brought a little present for you."

I opened my briefcase and took out a small machine, which I placed on the table between us. In my work with athletes and coaches, I had found this to be the clincher.

"What's that?" asked Mike.

"It's called a ZEO machine. You put it on your nightstand and wear this wireless headband to bed. By measuring and recording brain waves, it will record how long it took you to fall asleep, how many times you woke up during the night, what stages of sleep you experienced, and how long you slept overall. In the morning, it'll even provide you with a sleep score, so you can gauge how you did. Athletes really enjoy that aspect of it."

"Cool! How accurate is it?"

"Not as accurate as going to a sleep lab where technicians attach about 15 electrodes to your body, but it's pretty good. Plus, it comes with a jump drive so you can share your data with me over the Internet. Start recording tonight, then send me the results after two weeks. I'll review them and get back to you."

"Awesome! So this is like my own portable sleep coach?"

"Pretty much. You know, most people tend to overestimate how much sleep they get by almost 45 minutes. This device makes it totally objective. It's like using a bathroom scale to gauge how your weight-loss efforts are going."

"Professor, I gotta say this is way better than I expected. I'm so stoked I almost want to skip tonight's game, go back to my room right now, and get started. I can't thank you enough."

"Whoa now, don't go getting too excited. I want to see you play tonight and beat up on those Sabres."

"You got it, Professor. You can pick up those tickets at the Will Call window. It was great seeing you, and I'll be in touch."

And with that he delivered one more crushing handshake and walked off, already seeming a bit more energetic.

The Three Golden Rules of Sleeping to Win

1. Get your body's required amount of sleep every night.

2. Stick to a regular sleep-wake schedule every night.

3. Get your sleep in one continuous block.

Your Personal Sleep Coach

For more information about the ZEO Sleep Manager, visit http://www.myzeo.com/sleep/

Secrets of the Night

To: mGreenza@nhl.org
From: jbm@powersleep.org
RE: Review of data and suggestions

Dear Mike,

It was great seeing you in Buffalo a couple weeks ago, and thanks again for those tickets. It was a real thrill watching you play. I've reviewed the two weeks of data you sent. It looks like you're getting more sleep, you've established a fairly regular sleep-wake schedule, and you're sleeping in a less fragmented way. Hopefully, you're feeling the positive effects of this. However, your scores are not as high as I'd like to see, so let me make a few additional suggestions.

First, you're still not getting as much overall sleep as you should be. (Remember that someone your age needs 7½ to 8½ hours per night, compared to when you were in college and needed 9¼.) Also, you're not getting enough Stage 4 deep sleep and REM sleep. To help you understand why these stages are particularly important to athletes, let me briefly review what a great night's sleep should look like. This gets a bit technical, so just make believe you're back in one of my classes.

A healthy sleeper usually drifts off in 15 to 20 minutes. Your data shows you're typically falling asleep much faster than that, so this tells me you're still sleep-deprived. Try either moving up your bedtime or pushing back your wake time by 30 minutes.

Now, as you may recall, sleep can basically be divided into REM (rapid eye movement) and non-REM components. REM is the period in which most dreams (like winning the Stanley Cup) occur. Non-REM, which is also known as "slow-wave sleep," is subdivided into several stages, each with distinct brainwaves and purposes.

As you're closing your eyes and becoming relaxed, your brainwaves get slower and more regular. As you drift off, you enter Stage 1, where slow theta waves dominate brain activity and muscles further relax. The transition into Stage 2 is marked by a complete disengagement from the environment and is regarded by researchers as the true beginning of sleep. Next come Stages 3 and then 4 – the deepest sleep of the night. During these delta-wave stages, blood pressure drops, respiration slows, and blood flow to muscles decreases. For athletes, this slow-wave sleep is critical because it's when the secretion of human growth hormone (HGH) peaks. As you know, this stimulates muscle development and tissue repair.

After 30 to 40 minutes in Stage 4, you retrace your steps through Stages 3 and 2. However, instead of returning to Stage 1, your sympathetic nervous system becomes more active than it is even when awake.

Blood flow to the brain, respiration, pulse rate, blood pressure and body temperature all increase. Your eyes dart back and forth under their lids, and you enter REM sleep. This is when the previous day's experiences are solidified into memory. And here's the key: This includes muscle memory. So everything you worked on in practice? This is where it comes together.

It takes approximately 90 minutes to cycle through all these stages one time. When you're sleeping adequately, you'll visit REM four or five times during the night, with each period being twice as long as the last. That's why it's vital for athletes to get the recommended amount. If you cut even an hour of sleep, you're missing a huge portion of REM.

Mike, if these aren't reasons enough to keep working on this, something else happens in Stage 2–but only after about 6 ½ hours of sleep. We see the appearance of sleep spindles, triggering a cascade of calcium into the brain's motor cortex. This lays down even more lasting muscle memory for step-by-step sequences and quick, subconscious recall. Can you imagine thinking through every movement involved in a slap-shot? By the time you did that, someone would have stolen the puck. So practice your slap-shot and then get at least eight hours of sleep. By the next day it will be in your permanent motor-muscle memory. Without adequate sleep, what you work so hard on learning in practice is lost.

Got all that? Great!

Now here are just a few more pointers for sleeping better. They're little things, but they can make a big difference:

Make sure the bedroom is quiet, dark, and cool (somewhere between 65 and 67 degrees is ideal).

Keep bedroom clutter to a minimum and try to reserve the room only for sleeping. I know that's not possible in hotels, but at home keep the computer and television out.

Avoid caffeine after 2 p.m. Caffeine has a half-life of six hours, which means that six hours after your last sip, half the caffeine is still in your body. Warning: The majority of fast-food chains serve "decaf" coffee that actually contains up to nine times the amount of caffeine that a non-caffeinated beverage is supposed to (3 mg per 8 oz of water). And don't forget that chocolate and many energy drinks and sodas contain caffeine as well.

Don't consume any alcohol within three hours of bedtime. Research shows that alcohol interferes with, and can even destroy, critical stages of sleep that have a huge bearing on athletic performance.

Cut out all nicotine, and this includes smokeless tobacco. Nicotine is an even stronger stimulant than caffeine; it keeps you awake at night because your body is craving more.

Have a good-quality mattress at home so when you lie down your head, neck, and spinal cord are aligned just as if you were standing. This requires a high coil count (above 400 for queen- and 480 for king-size) innerspring mattresses, or a thick vinyl (above 20 mil) for waterbeds. If the mattress in your hotel room is shot, ask to either change rooms or have it replaced.

Test your pillow by folding it in half. If it opens instantly then it's providing adequate support. If it stays closed, it's dead. Either buy a new one or, if you tend to attract unwanted visitors, put it in the guest room! Once you find a pillow you love–and there are ones made to match every sleeping style (side, back, stomach…)–take it on the road with you. A company called Eagle Creek makes reusable Compression Sacs for travel that enable you to squeeze all the air out of a pillow so it takes up practically zero space in your suitcase.

Limit the use of electronics an hour before bed. The blue spectrum light these devices emit blocks the release of melatonin, the hormone that facilitates sleep. This includes TVs, computers, iPads and even mobile phones and tablet readers such as Nooks and Kindles. If that's too big a sacrifice, buy a pair of blue spectrum blocking glasses for use at that time.

Come up with some activities that help you de-stress and get to sleep quicker. Listen to some soothing music, try meditation, or just write your worries on a piece of paper to get them out of your head.

Finally, establish a nightly sleep routine. Just as a pre-game routine helps you get in the proper mindset, so will this. Have a low-protein/high-carb snack, take a hot bath, Jacuzzi or shower, do some light stretching, dim the bedroom lights…. Wherever you are, having a routine like this will help you get to sleep quicker and stay there.

That'll do it, Mike. Try to implement as many of these suggestions as you can, and continue using the ZEO monitor. I know this is a lot but trust me, it'll pay off. I guarantee you'll see a big difference in your energy level, your focus and, most important, your performance on the ice.

All the best from your sleep coach,

Jim

What Happens When the Lights Go Out

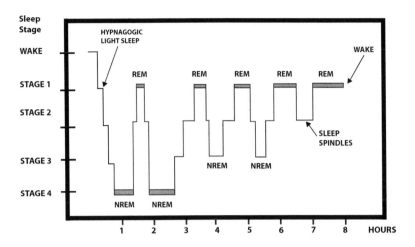

Fig. 1 shows the architecture of a good night's sleep. The dark blocks represent your time spent in REM sleep. Each REM cycle should be longer than the previous. Therefore, your sleep between hours seven and eight are critical for memory and athletic performance.

4 Teenage Walking Zombies

To: jbm@powersleep.org
From: mGreenza@nhl.org
RE: My little sister

Dear Prof,

Britt, who I mentioned to you awhile back, is not letting me forget that it was her idea to contact you. In fact, she's been pestering me to ask for some additional advice. She's a high-school freshman and will be trying out for the cross-country team this fall. Since she's pretty competitive, just like me, and will be up against much older girls, she's wondering if any of the tips you've already supplied could benefit her. I hate to infringe on any more of your time because you've already been so kind, but since your advice is working so well for me, I feel I owe it to her. Can you help?

Thanks,

Mike

To: mGreenza@nhl.org
From: jbm@powersleep.org
RE: My little sister

Mike,

I think one of the reasons zombies have become so popular lately among young people is because they remind them of themselves. Teenagers, and teen athletes in particular, are often so sleep-deprived they look and act like the walking dead.

All kidding aside, there's no need to apologize about asking for additional advice for Britt. This is what I do and, as you'll no doubt remember from class, I can go on endlessly about it! Everything we've discussed so far applies to your little sister except for one important thing: the amount of sleep someone between puberty and about age 26 requires on a nightly basis.

Sleep is a tricky issue for teens because there's a battle raging inside their bodies. Their need for sleep is higher than yours or mine because of all the physical and psychological development they're undergoing but, at the same time, it's usually harder for them to get to bed at a decent hour.

Research indicates that the teenage brain is biologically set to fall asleep at 3 a.m. and begin awakening at 11 a.m. Because schools start early in the morning, and many coaches call even earlier-morning practices, 80 percent of teens don't get enough sleep, and 43 percent confess to feeling tired all day. The fact that most teens need the alarm-clock equivalent of Big Ben proves they're getting inadequate rest.

One reason why it may be so difficult for teens to nod off early is because the body's natural sleep-enhancing hormone (melatonin) is blocked by the growth hormone and isn't secreted until much later in the evening. Nonetheless, teens should try to go to bed as early as naturally possible. And establishing a nightly pre-bed ritual, just like I recommended for you, can help trick the body into feeling sleepier.

Sleeping extra on the weekend to make up for late nights and early starts during the week is not a solution. While any additional shut-eye is helpful, sleeping until noon on Saturday and Sunday is not the best way to recover. Such a yo-yo schedule throws a teenager's internal clock off even more. Like you, Britt should pick a reasonable bedtime and rising time and stick to it every day. And she should be limiting caffeine consumption in the same way you are.

Now here's the really important part: For full alertness and optimal athletic performance, Britt needs 9¼ hours of sleep nightly. If she makes sleep a priority, she'll start seeing the benefits within two or three days. She'll have more energy for training, which will lead to more strength and endurance and a greater chance of making the team. Plus, she'll be more efficient and effective at everything else in her life. It really is that simple.

If she's still skeptical, here are three young athletes that I've had the pleasure of working with that she might find inspirational:

Sarah Hughes: Olympic Gold Medalist
As a young teenager, Sarah was looking for an extra edge that would help her realize her Olympic figure-skating dreams. Like most teens, she was barely

sleeping 7 hours per night and had an irregular sleep-wake schedule. She was also drinking coffee to stay alert after getting up at 4:30 a.m. for practice, spending all day in school, and then practicing more in the afternoon. This two-a-day schedule, although traditional in many sports, is a sure sleep and performance thief.

So I devised a new kind of training program for her – one that required 9¼ hours of sleep every night, with consistent sleep and wake times, and of course far less caffeine. This assured she would get the sleep she needed for someone her age, including the all-important "sleep spindles" that occur only after at least 6½ hours of continuous sleep. These spindles trigger a cascade of calcium in the brain, which enhance motor-muscle memory. In other words, this is when Sarah's body and mind really learns all those fancy moves she was practicing.

The most challenging part, though, was convincing Sarah and her coach to forgo the early-morning practices. But they agreed to the experiment and, although she was an underdog at the 2002 Olympic Games, she came home with the gold medal.

Amber Way: A Real Sleeper

As a high school freshman in Michigan, Amber was not expected to contribute much as a varsity cross-country and track runner. (Sound familiar?) But after hearing me speak on the importance of sleep and athletic performance, she decided to significantly change her habits. She committed to getting 9¼ hours of sleep per night and following a consistent sleep-wake schedule, even on weekends. As a result, she broke four school records that season and won a silver medal at states.

Jon Michael McGrath II: World Caliber

To be a champion trap and skeet shooter, you have to consistently hit at least 490 out of 500 targets. At 16 years of age, Jon wasn't doing that despite lots of practice. After hearing me speak about the importance of sleep and athletic performance, he established a 9¼-hour per night sleep schedule and, within a week, saw his scores rise. As a member of the U.S. Shotgun Team, he has since won numerous national and world titles. Here's a note I received from his dad:

> "We cannot thank you enough. We are true believers in [your work]. You not only made a difference for a young USA Athlete, but it was Jon Michael's gold-medal win that put the United States on top of the medal count, edging out China in the 2011 World Cup competition in Sydney. Jon Michael is intently focused on the amount of sleep he receives during the competition season to achieve and maintain peak performance."

Feel free to pass this info along to Britt, Mike, and have her email or call me directly with any further questions.

Best,
Jim

To: jbm@powersleep.org
From: brittneverquits@hotmail.com
RE: Sleep stuff

Dear Professor Maas,

You rock! Thanks for helping out my big bro (he's way less crabby now) and me. Never realized I needed so much sleep, but what you say makes sense. I'm gonna commit to it like you suggest and see if I can drop those other zombies come spring! Thanks!

Britt

5 A Win-Win Situation

To: jbm@powersleep.org
From: mGreenza@nhl.org
RE: Can we coach Coach?

Dear Prof,

Thanks for helping Britt and for your continued work on my behalf. I really appreciate it. I've taken many of your suggestions to heart and, just like you promised, have seen improvements in focus, attitude, energy level, and I even scored a hat trick the other night! I've also gotten some of my teammates involved in our experiment. But there's still one big problem. Coach Harkwell is old school, and he doesn't think something as simple as sleep can help a professional hockey team improve.

I've tried talking to him about some of the things we've discussed, but he's not listening. And he's continuing to call early-morning practices, believing that working hard builds commitment and champions.

I respect Coach Harkwell a lot, but this long season just

seems to keep getting longer. I don't see how we're going to be able to have the energy to make a push for the playoffs in the coming months.

I know I've asked a lot of you already, but is there any way to get through to him?

Mike

To: mGreenza@nhl.org
From: jbm@powersleep.org
RE: Can we coach Coach?

Dear Mike,

I can't tell you how many times I've encountered the exact situation you've described. Getting coaches to pay attention to sleep is a tough challenge. Even in medical residency programs, little if any education is provided about the role of sleep in health and performance. So it's hardly surprising that athletic coaches are basically ignorant about it.

Here's what we do: I've attached a letter that you can give to Coach Harkwell. Over the years I've shared a similar version with several coaches, from Little League to the major leagues, in a variety of sports, and it has never failed to get their attention. Read it over and, if you think it'll help, feel free to pass it along.

Jim

Dear Coach Harkwell,

I had the good fortune of being a faculty advisor to our university's hockey team when Mike Greenza played here. It was a pleasure to not only work closely with Mike as a scholar athlete but also see him improve so much under your mentorship in the years since. As you know, Mike is the type of guy who strives to be the best, and that's why he approached me a few weeks ago asking about the relationship of sleep to athletic excellence. I shared some exciting new findings with him that apply directly to hockey players and athletes in general.

He asked me to share the most significant of these discoveries with you.

As a psychologist and sleep researcher for 44 years, I've come to believe that sleep is a magic ingredient for raising performance levels in even the most highly trained professional athletes. With the proper amount of sleep, a number of important things happen: glucose metabolism increases, resulting in more energy; cortisol levels decline, reducing stress; growth hormone levels increase, benefiting muscle and bone development; and cognition, reaction time, coordination and recovery speed all improve. Here's a quick review of the latest research:

A study of a Pac-10 men's basketball team[1] found significant improvement in numerous key areas after the players adopted a regular sleep schedule of at least 10 hours per night for five to seven weeks. Specifically, there was a 9 percent increase in free-throw conversions, a 9.2 percent increase in three-point conversions, faster sprint intervals and reaction times, and a boost in overall physical and mental health.

The researchers then did a follow up study with the Stanford women's tennis team, finding that 10 hours of sleep per night for five weeks resulted in faster sprint times, a 42% boost in hitting accuracy, and better overall performance.

A study[2] of Major League Baseball draftees found that the sleep-deprived were less likely to make the team than their well-rested counterparts. The attrition rate for all draftees studied was 37.5

percent, compared to 57 percent for the sleepy ones.

In the National Football League[3] sleepiness predicted players' draft value as well. Draftees with the highest measures of sleepiness had only a 38.5 percent chance of remaining on the original team, while their better-rested counterparts had a 56.3 percent chance of making it.

A study of MLB batting averages[4] showed that a player's biological clock has a significant impact on performance. When an athlete is naturally at the most-alert phase of his sleep-wake cycle, he hits better.

Sleep extension enables swimmers to have a 17% improvement in reaction times off the starting block.

In another study involving the body's internal clock and natural sleep-wake cycle,[5] it was found that the timing of football games affects how likely a team is to win. The performance of West Coast vs. East Coast teams during Monday Night Football (9 p.m. Eastern, 6 p.m. Pacific) was compared. West Coast teams won almost twice as often and by more points than their East Coast counterparts. Strength, flexibility, and reaction time all seem to peak later in the day, making the prime time for athletic performance between 6 and 9 p.m. Therefore, West Coast teams have an advantage when traveling east because their biological clocks are advanced by three hours.

Research has shown that sleep deprivation is responsible for 90 percent of overtraining injuries.[6] During certain stages of sleep, the body regenerates damaged tissue and replenishes depleted energy stores. It was clear that injured athletes had increased the intensity of their workouts too quickly without being fully recovered.

Sleep deprivation slows glucose metabolism up to 40 percent.[7] This results in significantly less available energy for an athlete. Lack of sleep also decreases the production of human growth hormone (HGH), which plays a key role in tissue repair and muscle recovery.

Slow-wave or deep sleep plays a primary role in recovery from physical exhaustion.[8] Runners who were studied before and after a marathon stayed in deep sleep the night following the race significantly longer than the night before. This suggests that the body uses slow-wave sleep as a recovery period relating to exercise and athletic performance.

Dr. Cheri Mah, a sleep researcher at Stanford University notes it is no accident that athletes like Lebron James, Michelle Wie, Roger Federer and Usain Bolt get at least ten hours of sleep while training and playing. She advises players to get good sleep before game day, take a 20 minute pre-game nap, and train during the time of day you will be competing.

As you can see, Coach, just a few simple adjustments to sleep patterns have produced some remarkable results. Recently, I've convinced several professional coaches like yourself in the NBA, NFL and NHL to prioritize sleep and educate their players about its importance. Many have even agreed to forego early-morning practices for a while to gauge for themselves the impact that additional rest has on performance. With the playoffs fast approaching, perhaps a little extra sleep is all your team needs to bring the Stanley Cup to Philadelphia.

I hope this information has been helpful. If you have any questions or would like to discuss this further, let me know.

Best regards,
James B. Maas, Ph.D.

6 The Dos & Don'ts of Power Napping

"Hello, this is Jim."

"Professor, it's Mike Greenza. I hope you don't mind, but I had to give you a call and tell you the good news. Coach Harkwell just announced he's cutting back on morning practices so we can get more rest. I can't believe you got through to him! The mood on the team is better already. I figure this should give everybody about two more hours of sleep per night."

"That's great, Mike! When I didn't hear back from him, I thought he just ignored my note. It'll be interesting to see how the team responds in the next few weeks. You're heading into a big home stand, right?"

"Yeah, so it's the perfect time to try this. Everybody's excited. But I have another question. You have time?"

"Shoot."

"How does napping fit into all this? Some guys on the team nap for hours before a night game, others just grab 20 or 30 minutes, and I usually don't nap at all. What's the research say?"

"Good question. I should have gone over that with you. There's a lot of new research in this area. I'll try to keep it brief, but if I start to run on just stop me. You know what the definition of a professor is, don't you?"

"Try me."

"Someone who talks in other people's sleep."

"Good one! Go on, I'm all ears."

"The key is whether you're getting adequate sleep at night. If you are then you won't have the urge to nap. If you aren't, then there are definitely right and wrong ways to do it. So the first step is deciding if you're getting enough sleep overall, and that's an easy thing to do. Do you get really tired after lunch? Do your eyelids feel like mini-dumbbells halfway through the afternoon? If so, then napping is a simple, healthful way to quickly boost alertness, concentration, productivity, creativity, mood, and performance.

"Although it has acquired a stigma of laziness in society, even Fortune 500 CEOs do it. In fact, a British study found that simply anticipating a nap is enough to lower blood pressure. For many people and athletes, it's replacing the Starbucks run as the new midday pick-me-up.

"This is all based in science, of course. Our bodies are programmed with what's called a 'biphasic sleep pattern.' This simply means we cycle through two periods of drowsiness every 24 hours. One is between 2 and 4 p.m., and the other is in the late evening before bed. So napping is a very natural and healthful thing to do.

"But as I said before there's a right and a wrong way to do it. And that's the second step. Depending on how much time you have, a nap of 20 minutes or one lasting 90 minutes will refresh you most. The shorter nap takes you through the first two stages of sleep while the longer one encompasses the entire five-stage sleep cycle and awakens you in the first stage of the next cycle.

"Tell me, Mike, have you ever experienced waking up from a nap feeling groggy, ornery, and more tired than when you laid down."

"Yeah, I always wondered what I was doing wrong."

"You most likely napped between 30 and 80 minutes and woke up in a deep-sleep stage. You should always set an alarm when you nap so you're sure to wake up in a lighter sleep stage and feel more refreshed.

"The ideal pre-game nap, assuming you need one, is 90 minutes because it will include some REM sleep. Studies show that even just a small amount of REM can boost motor-skill performance by 16 percent. But 90 minutes is a long time for busy people, so 20 minutes is what I recommend most because it's better than nothing. Basketball player Steve Nash says that napping every game day, whether you feel like it or not, has a positive effect on your performance that night and a cumulative effect on your body throughout the season."

"Now most nap-a-phobes assume there's no way they'll be able to relax, doze off, and derive any benefit from sleeping such a short time. But they're missing the point. A nap is not the same type of sleep experience you get at night. Think of it this way: Your body is hungry for sleep, but you can't give it a full-course meal during the day. So you provide a satisfying snack – one that replenishes energy stores, takes the edge off appetite, and allows you to continue functioning without distraction."

"That's a great analogy, Professor. I never thought of it that way."

"Good. So if you or any of your teammates want to try this, I would recommend starting with a 20-minute power nap. If that works and you have the time, try 90 minutes. Always set that alarm, though. As long as you don't have a history of insomnia, napping like this shouldn't interfere with your nighttime rest. In fact, some insomniacs find that napping reduces their anxiety about sleeping and actually helps them doze off more easily at night. Skipping naps when you're tired also doesn't help you sleep any better or longer at night. That's a common misconception."

"One more question, Professor. Do all the rules about sleeping well at night also apply to napping well?"

"Absolutely. You want to try to clear your mind as best you can of any 'nap blockers.' This can be as simple as doing some breathing exercises or just telling yourself that you'll deal with the demands of the day when you wake up in 20 or 90 minutes. Try to lie down so you won't jerk yourself awake as you start to fall asleep. You've trained your body to associate certain positions with sleep, so anything you can do to trick it into thinking it's bedtime will help."

"Put your mobile phone on silent and take any other necessary steps to minimize noise, such as using earplugs or noise-canceling headphones. Block out light as well, even if it means using an eye mask. And since naps occur when our core body temperature is highest, cooling the room is even more important than at night. Many people find that turning on an air conditioner or fan not only helps with this but also provides soothing ambient noise."

"Awesome stuff, Professor. I can't thank you enough."

"No problem, Mike. I'll type up a quick summary of these tips and email them to you, so you can share them with everyone. Can't wait to see how this all turns out for the team!"

8 Simple Steps to the Perfect Nap

1. Decide if you really need one. (If you're getting adequate nighttime rest—7½ to 9¼ hours—you shouldn't.)

2. Choose between 20 or 90 minutes. (Anything in between will leave you feeling worse.)

3. Set a dependable alarm.

4. Eliminate disturbing noise by wearing earplugs or turning on something that generates ambient sound (i.e., air conditioner, fan, radio set between stations...).

5. Block light by pulling shades or wearing an eye mask.

6. Cool the room to 65-68 degrees Fahrenheit.

7. Lie down. (Trying to nap while sitting in an unsupported position keeps muscles from fully relaxing.)

8. Clear your mind as best you can.

7

Winning Ways When You're Away

During the next few weeks, the Flyers won seven of eight, and Mike scored five goals. I have to admit, for an old professor who's been at this a very long time it was pretty exciting. When I couldn't watch the games on TV, I had score alerts sent to my phone. It was like one giant lab experiment, with exceedingly positive results.

Mike emailed me regularly. His ZEO scores were right on target, and some of his teammates had even ordered sleep monitors of their own. And Coach Harkwell had actually heeded my advice and didn't schedule any early-morning practices. The team was finally starting to gel.

But the real test was coming up. The Flyers would be traveling for the next few weeks on the longest road trip of the season. If there was ever a time when all our progress could be derailed, this was it. A succession of night games followed by midnight flights through various time zones… these guys were heading into the perfect storm of sleep deprivation and athletic performance. Even I was worried.

So I wasn't too surprised to get an email from Coach Harkwell himself a few days before the team was scheduled to leave….

To: jbm@powersleep.org
From: wharkwell@nhl.org
Re: Road Trip

Dear Dr. Maas,

It's Will Harkwell. Sorry I didn't respond to your previous email, but I knew Mike was keeping you posted, and I figured you were following our progress on the sports pages.

I've been coaching for more than 20 years, and I never really considered that my morning practices might be harming my players. I appreciate your taking the time to educate me. The information you provided is making me reconsider other aspects of our program and how we train our athletes. Once the season is over, we should get together to discuss all of this in depth. But for now I have a pressing question that I hope you can answer.

As you know, we've been playing pretty well lately and, I believe, we have a genuine shot at winning our division if we keep it up. But this next road trip is a West Coast swing, and it's going to be one of the most brutal I've ever experienced:

Sunday - fly to Winnipeg
Monday - play in Winnipeg, fly to Dallas that night getting in at 4am
Tuesday - Practice day
Wednesday - Play Dallas at night, fly to Washington, getting in at 3am
Thursday - practice day
Friday - play in Washington, fly to Philadelphia, getting in at 1am

How the hell am I going to keep these kids well-rested and on top of their game when we're playing in 3 cities in 6 days and covering a total of 6,800 miles?

Any advice you can provide will be greatly appreciated.

Regards,

Will Harkwell
Head Coach
Philadelphia Flyers

To: wharkwell@nhl.org
From: jbm@powersleep.org
Re: Road Trip

Dear Coach Harkwell,

I'm glad you're becoming a believer in sleeping to win, and I'm happy to help in any way I can. You're wise to be worried about this upcoming trip. Jet lag is one of the biggest and most frustrating obstacles that traveling athletes face. Fortunately, there's some new research and strategies for how to deal with it. Let me provide a quick review, along with some suggestions on what you can do.

First, you need to understand what occurs physiologically during travel across time zones. Jet lag is really nothing more than the de-synchronization of the body's natural circadian rhythm. More simply, it's when our internal biological clock no longer matches the one on the wall where we're located. So when the team travels from Philadelphia to Winnipeg on the first leg of the trip, all the chemical regulators in your player's bodies will be on East Coast time. For most people, this is an inconvenience that works itself out in a few days. But for athletes who are expected to perform at a high level soon after arrival, it has significant effects. On the ice, jet lag results in less endurance, power and alertness. Players fatigue more easily and make more mental mistakes. But its impact doesn't stop there. It extends beyond the ice into everyday life, inhibiting digestion, thinking, motivation, concentration and mood. And it all compounds the more you travel.

So when exactly does jet lag occur? Although any kind of long-distance travel is tiring, this de-synchronization of our body clocks generally only happens when two or more time zones are crossed. Additionally, traveling east is worse than going west. That's because our clocks actually run on a 25-hour cycle, making us want to naturally draw out our days. When traveling west, we just need to stay awake a few extra hours, so it's not that big a deal. But traveling in the opposite direction is more difficult because we have to force ourselves to sleep sooner.

Sorry for the long-winded explanation. I'm a professor, after all. So here's what I recommend you do:

>Leave immediately after your last home game. You won't get to Winnipeg until the wee hours of the morning, everyone will be exhausted, and that will not give the team enough days to adjust. The general rule is to allow the body one day of adjustment for every time zone crossed. So since you're going from Philly to Winnipeg, you'll not be in great shape. When a crazy travel schedule doesn't meet this requirement, tell the guys to sleep on the plane and upon arrival let them sleep in until noon. Forget the morning skate! I know it's violating my rule of a regular sleep-wake schedule, but being sleep deprived is worse than maintaining a rigid schedule in the short run. Incidentally, we are encouraging the leagues in all sports to be ever mindful of jet lag when planning the season's schedule. It will benefit the players, the quality of competition, and reduce injuries. Meanwhile, my advice is to get sleep whenever possible, day or night.

>If that's not possible, begin adjusting your players' schedules to the destination's time zone a few days before leaving. Move any practices up by an hour and encourage them to similarly adjust their sleeping and eating habits. This shouldn't affect their performance

at home, but it will make adapting to West Coast time easier once they arrive.

>It's crucial that your players be well-rested before leaving on this road trip, so I definitely would not schedule any early-morning practices or team meetings. In fact, if there are any outside events or media commitments for the early a.m., I would try to cancel them. Any outstanding sleep debt that your players owe their bodies beforehand will be exaggerated by the change in time.

>In addition to these steps, consider using what's called "light exposure therapy" to help speed up the adjustment of your players' biological clocks. This method, combined with the strategy I've laid out, is the most effective way to beat jet lag. For each guy on the team, you can purchase a device called a Litebook. It's portable, costs about $175, and emits "bright daylight spectrum light." Because our bodies rely on external cues like the sun to tune our internal clocks, this device works great. I've recommended it successfully to many other athletes and teams. Here's how it's used:

--Sit down, turn the device on, and set it 2 feet away and at a 45-degree angle to your face. (Do not look directly at the light.) Then simply read, eat, watch TV, or work at a computer for 15 to 20 minutes.

--When traveling west, use the device in the afternoon to extend the day. When heading east, use it on the flight when it's nighttime in your body but already daytime at your destination.

--Even when you're in the midst of a home stand, exposure to this type of light can boost alertness.

Consider it a secret weapon if any of your players miss some sleep and feel drowsy before a game. Or, use it in the locker room just before taking the ice for a game scheduled between 2 p.m. and 4 p.m., which is when we naturally experience a dip in alertness.

> Before departing, encourage your players to bring their pillows from home to use on the plane and in the hotels. During the flight, recommend drinking plenty of water and avoiding the dehydrating effects of alcohol. Have them use noise-canceling headphones to reduce the fatiguing effect of engine noise, too.

>Obviously, if it's bedtime when the team is flying everyone should try to get some sleep. Since most of us are usually sleep-deprived, it's not a bad idea to use travel time to repay any sleep debt so don't hesitate to take a good nap.

>After arriving at your destination, encourage your players to spend some time outdoors. Exposure to natural sunlight is the most effective way to sync their body clocks. If that's not possible, at least encourage them to open the drapes in their hotel rooms.

>Emphasize to everyone that caffeine after 2 p.m. or alcohol within three hours of bedtime interferes with sleep and should be avoided, especially before a game. In fact, you might want to consider banning both on certain flights. Educate your players, too, about the use of energy drinks and smokeless tobacco. Most don't realize how much of a stimulant these are. In fact, the reason they're probably using them in the first place is to compensate for a lack of sleep. So it's a vicious circle they need to break if they're ever going to make progress.

>High-intensity exercise should be avoided the day of arrival so as not to amplify the results of travel fatigue. Notice, however, that I said "high-intensity." A loosen-up skate or some other low-key effort is fine and, some studies show, may even be helpful in counteracting jet lag.

>Have your team manager do his or her research and book hotels with soundproof rooms. Many hotels these days are also offering "sleep menus" that include different mattress and pillow options. The perfect sleep environment is cool, dark and quiet. You can follow all my suggestions, but if the hotel is Party Central then all is lost.

>Finally, when you have an important game coming up, focus on the sleep your team gets two nights prior. A study published in the Journal of Sports Medicine and Physical Fitness found that the quantity and quality of sleep on this night was more influential on aerobic performance than the one immediately prior to the event. So the old coach's adage of, "Get a good night's sleep because we have a big game tomorrow" should be amended to, "Get a good night's sleep because we have a big game in two days."

That's the best information and advice I have, Coach. Hope it helps. And, of course, if you have any other questions, let me know.

Good luck!

Jim Maas

8 Sleep Thieves: Drugs and Alcohol

To: jmb@powersleep.org
From: mGreenza@nhl.org
Re: Party!?

Dear Prof,

Just a quick note to say it's been a great road trip so far. We're playing our best hockey of the season and, as you probably know, we're the hottest team in our conference right now. The puck actually seems like it's traveling in slow motion for me. I'm seeing, anticipating, shooting and skating better than ever. It's unbelievable the effect that your advice has had, not just on me but the entire team.

As usual, though, I have another question. With all this newfound success, we're the center of attention. Girls, reporters, old friends…everyone wants to hang out with us. And the guys and I naturally want to enjoy it all and celebrate. I know you told Coach Harkwell and me that alcohol interferes with sleep and should be avoided entirely the night before a game, but given all the other things we're doing to improve our sleep habits, is it really that important? Can't we have just a little fun (within reason, of course)?

Mike

To: mGreenza@nhl.org
From: jbm@powersleep.org
Re: Party!?

Hi Mike,

Thanks for checking in! Two games out of playoff contention with less than a month left in the season? I better get in line for playoff tickets! But at the risk of sounding like, well, your old professor, the biggest mistake you guys can make right now is celebrating too soon. Not only will overconfidence mess up your heads, but the partying that results will put you right back where you were in November – sleep-deprived and at the bottom of your division.

A former student of mine, Hayley Hughes, is an expert on the detrimental effects of drugs and alcohol on athletic performance. In fact, she's more up-to-date on that research than I. So if you don't mind, I'm going to forward your email to her so she can respond directly. I think you'll find what she has to say very interesting.

All the best,

Professor Jim

To: mGreenza@nhl.org
From: hayley19@powersleep.org
Re: Party!?

Hi Mike,

Dr. Maas asked me to update you on the latest research concerning the effects of alcohol and other drugs on athletic performance. I'm aware of your growing reputation on the ice. As a former college hockey player myself (on a national women's championship team, I might add immodestly), I'm a big fan of the sport. So I know the temptations you're facing, especially when on the road. I realize you asked specifically about alcohol, but I hope you don't mind if I run through some other drugs commonly used by athletes and the misconceptions surrounding them. I think you and your teammates will find it helpful:

Nicotine: Many athletes in all sports have come to believe that nicotine is a performance enhancer. Even though they would never smoke a cigarette for health reasons, they depend on a little chew to get them up for games and supposedly play better. However, there's no significant scientific evidence that this is true. Although nicotine is a stimulant that delivers a mild energy boost, there's no definitive proof that it sharpens focus or coordination.[1] Any benefits that seem to result probably stem from the dependency itself. In other words, the boost you feel after putting a pinch between your cheek and gum is your body shrugging off withdrawal symptoms. And if you happen to play better, it's simply because you expect to on a little nicotine.

I'm not going to launch into a long lecture (I'll save those for Professor Maas!) about the health effects of chronic tobacco use. Everyone knows its impact on the heart and other body parts. But there are a few other effects that are less well known and directly impact athletes like yourself. Over time, chronic nicotine use has been shown to actually decrease cognitive performance[1] or, in your case, the ability to stay alert, shoot or pass with accuracy, and maintain split-second reaction times. And as I'm sure Dr. Maas has mentioned, nicotine users are two times more likely to sleep poorly than non-users.

Since nicotine is so addictive, quitting isn't easy. In fact, withdrawal symptoms can include insomnia, anxiety, depression, irritability and poor concentration.[1] These can last several weeks. Therefore, it's probably best for any of your teammates with this problem to wait until after winning the Stanley Cup (think positive!) to stop completely.

Marijuana: Although illegal, it is an unfortunate reality that some athletes report using marijuana recreationally and/or to help them sleep or play better. However, THC, the main psychoactive component of the cannabis plant, has been shown to decrease the amount and quality of REM sleep.[2,3,4] Impeding REM sleep (including during a withdrawal period) can have an effect on brain cell growth, memory, learning of complex tasks, hormone secretions, muscle and bone growth. The effects of marijuana on Stage 4 sleep and total slow wave sleep have been inconsistent. One study showed that any helpful effects of the drug to induce sleep were less common after multiple years of use.[5] A short-term solution may in fact be a long term problem for your health. This issue is especially salient when stopping chronic marijuana use. Many people have withdrawal symptoms that can negatively affect sleep (e.g., less slow wave sleep and worse sleep efficiency).[6]

You or your teammates may feel quite tired and less energized in the morning, since THC is eliminated from your body quite slowly.[7] Therefore, your energy level may not be at the level you want it during your morning skate, run, or lift. I recommend finding a healthier (and legal) way to fall asleep, and I'm sure Dr. Maas has been doing his best to bring you up to speed on the best way to do that!

Caffeine: Unlike nicotine, caffeine is a proven performance enhancer.[8,9] It sharpens focus and even frees up fatty acids in the bloodstream to fuel endurance exercise. But both Dr. Maas and I believe these advantages are not worth the tradeoff – namely the disruption of sleep that results. Caffeine after 2 p.m., whether it's a cup of coffee, an energy drink, or even a piece of post-game chocolate cake, will likely keep you up and/or limit your time in deep restorative sleep. Keep in mind that many sports drinks and gels have caffeine (read the labels carefully!), as do some coffee brands that are advertised as decaf. So while it's okay to have a Starbucks in the morning or an energy drink before practice, respect that 2 p.m. cut-off. In fact, with the proper rest the need for caffeine should naturally diminish.

Adderall: This is a prescription drug used to treat attention deficit hyperactivity disorder. It has a calming effect in people with that condition. However, if you don't have ADHD, it acts as a powerful stimulant, perhaps improving mental performance and combating fatigue, including jet lag. This is why its use among the general population and athletes in particular has expanded in recent years. Although these effects may sound tempting, Adderall can create serious physical and psychological dependencies (it's in the same chemical class as amphetamine) while adversely impacting the cardiovascular system. Side effects include nervousness, restlessness, headache, uncontrollable shaking of a part of the body, difficulty sleeping, difficulty staying asleep, nausea, stomach pain, dry mouth, diarrhea, weight loss, pounding or fast heartbeat, shortness of breath, excessive tiredness, seizures, weakness in the arms or legs, dizziness, chest pain, paranoia, and blurred vision. Again, its possible performance-enhancing effects just aren't worth it.

Alcohol: Clearly, drinking has all the immediate effects (slower reaction time, decreased coordination…) and long-range consequences (nutritional deficiencies, muscle wasting, testosterone decline…) that athletes want to avoid. But it's certainly a great way to beat stress, relax, and celebrate another victory. You asked whether Dr. Maas's recommendation for avoiding alcohol the night before a game could be relaxed given all the other things you're doing to improve your sleep patterns. That's a good question. But the answer – if winning and optimal performance is still your priority – is a definitive "no." Here's why:

First, drinking beer is not a good way to replace carbohydrates after a game, as many athletes believe. Those post-game brews actually decrease the synthesis and storage of muscle glucose, so the next day your body has less of its main energy source available.[10] That lack of glucose impairs performance. Beer also doesn't re-hydrate the body. Instead, it dehydrates it even further, which is why you wake up thirsty in the middle of the night. And if you drink too much, the ensuing hangover will decrease your aerobic capacity and cloud your thinking the following day.[10]

Since your body is in recovery mode after a game, you may also be reducing its ability to soothe inflammation and soreness, which can make you more susceptible to injury. Drinking regularly also weakens the immune system,[11] so you may get sick more often. And as I'm sure Dr. Maas has already explained, any alcohol within three hours of bedtime will disturb REM sleep, which is critical for athletic performance, and interfere with other aspects of rest, if only because you'll need to get up to pee more frequently.

So the bottom line is that you don't have to become a teetotaler, you just have to be smart about when and how much you indulge. Here are three tricks I learned when I was playing hockey: 1) Re-hydrating immediately after a game reduces the urge to guzzle beer later simply because you're not as thirsty; 2) Light beer contains significantly less alcohol than regular beer, so it's not as dehydrating IF you limit yourself to one or two, and; 3) There's nothing wrong with ordering a non-alcoholic beer or a club soda if the real reason you're out on the town is for the social benefits. Try it. People may even respect you more for it.

Sex: Many athletes wonder how sex affects performance and, since it can become a sort of drug to some, I'll address it as well. Unless you stay up all night before a game, there's no evidence that sex weakens muscles, creates undue fatigue, or negatively impacts athletic performance in any way.[12] In fact, it may actually enhance it by promoting relaxation,[13,14] deeper sleep, and testosterone production,[15] which aids in aggressive sports like hockey. Some studies have even found that sex masks the pain of sports injuries.[16]

One important aspect that many athletes fail to consider, however, is the emotional impact of sex.

When a relationship sours, it can influence every other aspect of life including what you do on the ice. The resulting negativity and even hostility can create frustration and depression that manifests as a lack of motivation, energy, and concentration.[17] The resulting stress will also keep you up at night. To excel, athletes need to balance on a life wire that's neither too tight nor too relaxed. The level of tension is different for everyone. The key to walking that line successfully is anticipating all the little things that can knock you off balance.

Mike, I hope this helps. Feel free to share this information with your coach and teammates or email me with any further questions you may have. Keep playing great, and I'm rooting for you to reach the playoffs!

Best of luck,
Hayley Hughes

Alcohol Content of Various Beers

Type of Beer	% Alcohol	Calories (12 oz serving)
Bud Light	4.2	110
Budweiser	5.0	145
Michelob Ultra	4.1	95
Miller Genuine Draft "64"	2.8	64
Miller Lite	4.2	96
New Belgium Trippel	7.8	215
Pabst Blue Ribbon	4.7	144
Sam Adams Boston Lager	4.8	160
Sam Adams IPA	5.9	175
Sierra Nevada Pale Ale	5.6	175
Heineken Lager	5.4	150
Molson Canadian	5.1	144

Hidden Sources of Caffeine

Type of Drink/Food	Caffeine Amount (mg) in 8 oz Serving
Monster Energy Drink	80
Rockstar Energy Drink	80
Red Bull Energy Drink	80
Coffee (decaf, instant)	3
Coffee (decaf, brewed)	6
Starbucks Short Coffee	180
Dunkin Donuts Coffee	106
Tea (brewed)	47
Starbucks Tazo Earl Grey	65
Herbal Tea (brewed)	0
Diet Pepsi	24
Coca-Cola	23
Hershey's Milk Chocolate Bar	3 mg / 1.5 oz
Excedrin Migraine	130 mg / 2 caplets

9 Food for Thought

To: mGreenza@nhl.org
From: jbm@powersleep.org
cc: wsterling@eatwell.net
RE: Eat to Sleep

Hi Mike,

I hope Hayley's tips have made it clear why you really need to stay focused these next few weeks. Trust me, it'll pay off, and there will be plenty of time to celebrate after you win the Stanley Cup!

Since we're at such a crucial stage of the season, I want to share some nutritional advice with you. I know you already have an excellent team nutritionist, so I won't bore you with general diet advice. Rather, I want to share some little-known information about how certain foods and eating patterns affect sleep and athletic performance.

If you don't mind, I'd like to put you in touch with Wendy Sterling, whom I'm copying on this email. She's a nutritionist and a good friend, who has worked with the New York Jets and other high-profile athletes and teams. When I mentioned our "little experiment" the other day over lunch, she told me a few things that I believe can further help you. When you have a minute, just jot down a list of what (and when) you typically eat during the day and send it to her. This will help her pinpoint potential trouble spots. I'm sure you'll find what she has to say fascinating and useful.

Jim "Still Too Fat" Maas

To: mGreenza@nhl.org
From: wSterling@eatwell.net
RE: Eat to Sleep

Hi Mike,

It's great to meet you! Dr. Maas has told me so much about you. I appreciate your taking the time to send me your sample daily diet. As I expected, you're eating many of the right foods but the timing of those meals could be improved. Doing so will enhance the quality and quantity of sleep you're presently getting. So if you think you're playing well now, just wait!

I see that you eat your main meal pretty late – usually around midnight on game days. Then you skip breakfast, grab a high-protein lunch, and have a substantial snack in the late afternoon. Although you may not be noticing it, I think this eating schedule is disrupting your sleep pattern on some level and depriving you of even more energy and athletic benefits.

Think about this: Essentially, you're getting the bulk of your calories from one meal. You're dumping all this fuel into your body, asking your digestive system to process it (before bed, no less!), and then operating for much of the next day without fully replenishing your energy stores. Tell me, do you feel uncomfortable when you go to bed? Is the reason you're skipping breakfast because you're just not hungry? If so, these are signs you're eating too much at night.

I'd like to see the size of your meals become more consistent throughout the day. Because you can't eat any earlier on game days (two to three hours before bed would be ideal), I recommend you reduce the size of your late-night meal and then add a substantial breakfast followed by smaller "snack-meals" every three to four hours throughout the day. You should aim for most of your meals to be about 600-700 calories, meaning you'll probably have to start by shaving off about 200-300 cal at dinner right off the bat and then focus on making the rest of your meals about equal to that size. The first calories to eliminate are juices, sodas, caffeinated beverages, alcohol, and high sugar desserts.

Because your metabolism is still relatively high and you're burning so many calories with strenuous exercise, redistributing your food intake in this way will stabilize your energy level. Mood swings and lapses in concentration should disappear, plus you may experience an even deeper level of restful sleep – all of which will directly benefit your performance on the ice.

You might also discover you haven't been eating enough. Some athletes I've counseled with eating schedules similar to yours found they were actually "under-fueling." That's because eating one big meal late at night can trick the brain into thinking the body has eaten more throughout the day than it actually did. If you start waking up earlier than planned after adopting this new eating pattern then your blood glucose levels are dropping too low at night. Eat a little bit more throughout the day until this symptom goes away.

Another component that's equally important to a good night's rest is the kind of food you're ingesting in that last meal of the day. It can have a profound effect on how well you sleep. Specifically, you should avoid high-fat, high-fiber, and spicy foods. These can cause heartburn, acid reflux, coughing, and gas. Pizza, Mexican, Chinese, Indian, burgers, fries…these are all sleep disruptors when eaten before bed. High-fat food not only makes us feel uncomfortable but it also takes longer to digest. And although high-level athletes like yourself need extra sodium to replace what's sweated out, any salty foods, such as anchovy pizza, should be avoided before bed because you'll wake up with a powerful thirst.

For your last meal of the day, it's smarter to choose a turkey sandwich with hummus, a chicken breast with a baked potato, some pasta with a mild sauce, or a tofu-and-veggie stir-fry. In other words, opt for the bland and easily digestible, especially post-game. And definitely pass on all the usual sugary desserts. These will crank you up when you should be winding down.

Likewise, there are certain food ingredients that can facilitate sleep. You've probably joked about how tryptophan is responsible for knocking out your entire family after Thanksgiving dinner. Believe it or not, there is scientific proof of this. Tryptophan is an amino acid that induces sleepiness. It's present in turkey, nuts, seeds, bananas, eggs, and milk. In fact, many athletes find a bowl of healthful cereal to be an ideal dessert, late-night snack, or even meal. On those nights when you don't have a game, I suggest eating dinner earlier (say 6 or 7 p.m.) and then having a 100- to 300-calorie snack built from any of these tryptophan-rich foods an hour before bed.

People also tend to have personal "soothe foods." These are usually associated with fond childhood memories and help us relax. For instance, chamomile tea is a popular nightcap (although there's still no definitive proof it promotes sleep). Think about your own comfort food and, as long as it's not mom's meatloaf, feel free to use it to unwind before bed if it's convenient.

I know that Dr. Maas and his colleague have been warning you about the sleep-disrupting effects of alcohol and caffeine, so I won't belabor that. But here's one thing you may not know: Alcohol also promotes fat storage, hence the proverbial "beer gut." As you age and your natural speed and reaction time begins to fade, the last thing you want is to be carrying extra weight that will further slow you down. And, along the same lines, be wary of all the energy foods and drinks that companies probably bombard you with. Many are high in calories, sugar, caffeine, and ingredients whose healthfulness may be questionable. Although some of these products have their place in an athlete's diet for special circumstances, always read the labels and never ingest any of them before bed.

Finally, because your schedule is so crazy and you travel so much, I realize that maintaining a healthful diet, let alone one that promotes quality sleep, is probably one of your greatest challenges. But my experience with other athletes has shown that what I've outlined here is doable. All it takes is committing to the importance of nutrition in much the same way you've already done for sleep and simply tweaking your eating schedule to more equitably distribute daily calorie intake.

I hope this helps, Mike. Let me know if you have any questions, and good luck with the rest of the season!

Best regards,
Wendy Sterling, MD, RD, CSSD, CDN

Best/Worst Bedtime Snacks

EAT:

- ☑ Fiber and whole grains

- ☑ Crackers

- ☑ Sparkling water

- ☑ 2 tbsp hummus with vegetables

- ☑ Banana, apple

- ☑ Dried fruit and nuts

- ☑ Peanut butter, almond butter

- ☑ Cereals, oats

AVOID:

- ☒ Alcohol

- ☒ Caffeine (chocolate)

- ☒ Spicy food

- ☒ Dairy products (cheese, yogurt)

- ☒ Meats high in protein (sausage)

- ☒ Processed food or MSG

- ☒ Garlic

10

Injury, Recovery & Sleep

"Hello, Jim Maas speaking."

"Hey Prof, it's Mike!"

"Mike! Great job last weekend! You guys are really going great guns."

"You said it. There are only two weeks left in the season, and we've nailed down a playoff berth. But that's not why I'm calling. Yesterday toward the end of practice I pulled a hamstring, and it looks like I'm going to be out a while. The doctors say it may take a few weeks to recover, and they already have me in rehab. But, honestly, I'm worried. I've never pulled a hammy this bad before. It even turned black-and-blue. I don't want to miss the playoffs and let the team down, but I know I'm going to lose fitness and, even if I can come back, I won't be at 100 percent."

"Sorry to hear that, Mike. I had no idea. There was nothing on the sports report this morning."

"Yeah, the team hasn't announced it yet. They're waiting for the final medical reports to come back."

"Tell me something, Mike. I'm curious. How were you sleeping before this happened? Any problems?"

"As a matter of fact, I was pretty tired. We just got back from another road trip, there's been the pressure to make the playoffs, plus my girlfriend and I recently broke up. So I haven't exactly been sleeping like a baby lately. Why? Do you think there's some connection?"

"I do. Athletes often injure themselves in the final minutes of a workout or game. They may think it's because they're pushing real hard, but an underlying reason may be simple fatigue. You're tired, you're not as coordinated, your muscles may not have fully recovered from the last workout.... It definitely plays a role."

"Man, I had no idea. But, you're right, it makes total sense."

"Exactly. In fact, a couple of months ago, researchers looked at ACL injuries among NBA players[1]. They found that their fatigue levels correlated directly to when these injuries occurred. In a 48-minute game, the most damage was done between the 33rd and 39th minute – right when they were getting pretty tired. The thing is, it's not just physical exertion that brings on exhaustion, but also the fatigue that stems from poor sleep. When your body's tired, it's more susceptible to injury."

"Wow, sounds like I'm the perfect lab rat. I won't make that mistake again. But here's what I really want to know and the reason why I'm calling. Since sleep seems to fix so many things, I'm wondering if adjusting how much I'm getting or even when I'm getting it might actually help me heal this injury faster."

"Mike, the good news is that it definitely can. The relationship between exertion and injury that I just described works both ways. The more sleep you get, the more efficiently and effectively you'll recover. A number of studies have been done to demonstrate sleep's role in athletic recovery. Remember when I told you about sleep labs, where they hook you up to all sorts of electrodes to monitor your brain waves?"

"Yeah, you said that was the gold standard."

"Well, when researchers monitored the brain waves of runners on the nights before and after a marathon, they discovered they had more slow-wave sleep following the race.[2] This shows the body's natural need for this type of sleep to facilitate recovery. As I explained before, slow-wave sleep is the deepest of the night, and it's vital for athletes because this is when human growth hormone is secreted, which stimulates muscle development and tissue repair."

"So are you saying my hammy needs more slow-wave sleep in particular? And if so, how do I get that?"

"Fortunately, it's pretty easy. Slow-wave sleep is critical, but overall REM sleep is important, too. You need both. The key is to make sure to get enough total sleep every night. Your body runs on what's called a 'sleep homeostat,' meaning it regulates how much of each type of sleep it needs. It's like an auto-pilot mechanism, making all the necessary adjustments in your sleep course without you even knowing it. As long as you're getting enough total hours of shuteye, your body will work out the specifics. So stick with a consistent sleep schedule and let yourself wake up naturally in the morning, which means no alarm clocks or wake-up calls. And when you are sick due to a cold, flu or even a bad meal, get as much extra sleep as you can."

"What about my physical therapy sessions? Some start at 8:30 a.m., and my trainer is insisting I need to be at all of them if I'm going to heal quickly."

"I agree – you don't want to skip any of them, but waking up early for therapy is no different than waking up early for practice. Sleep is the priority. Try to explain that to him, or send me his email and I'll explain why pushing your sessions back to late morning or even early afternoon will hasten the whole recovery process even more."

"If this works, I'm gonna have to start calling you Doc rather than Prof! Thanks for the advice. I'll make it happen."

"Oh Mike, one more thought. The most important thing to remember is to let your body fully recover before you start skating again. I know you're anxious to be at full strength for the playoffs, but these final games don't really mean anything because you've already secured a berth. Although no injury is a good injury, if one was going to happen this was probably the best time. You have two weeks to play it smart. Many studies have been done on the tendency for athletes to hurry recovery and nearly every one shows that inadequate rest at such a critical time can lead to muscle damage, inflammation, and other problems. It's been a long season, and you've made a lot of progress. This might just be a case of your body saying it needs a little rest. If you give it what it needs, you may find this injury was actually a blessing in disguise."

11

Giving Nature a Nudge

To: jbm@powersleep.org
From: mGreenza@nhl.org
RE: Sleep Aids

Dear Doc,

Sorry I've been out of touch lately but, as I'm sure you know, I'm back on the ice and feeling stronger than ever. Although that hamstring pull scared the heck out of me, it *was* a blessing in disguise. It helped me get better rested physically and better prepared psychologically for the playoffs. Sweeping the first round was a big confidence booster for the team and me.

But now we're really up against it. We drew Boston in the semis, and the Bruins have been our nemisis all year. There's enormous pressure on us to win, and I already have butterflies the size of pterodactyls in my stomach. In fact, the entire team is on edge about this series. Since you taught us the importance of getting proper rest, we're worried we'll be unable to continue to do so given all the stress. There's even been talk in the locker room about using sleeping pills. What do you think about that? Is it a good idea?

Thanks,
Mike

To: mGreenza@nhl.org
From: jbm@powersleep.org
RE: Sleep Aids

Dear Mike,

You better believe I've been following you! In fact, I subscribed to NHL GameCenter LIVE so I won't miss a minute of the playoffs. I practically never leave the house!

I understand the pressure you must be facing, and it's normal to be concerned about losing sleep during such a time. Stress-induced insomnia – that's the official name – can have significant negative effects on athletic performance, regardless of the heightened motivation and adrenaline you're experiencing. I'm going to ask a former teaching assistant of mine, Maura Greenwood, to respond to your concern. She's now a clinical psychologist who specializes in treating sleep disorders. She'll fill you in on the advantages and disadvantages of the most common sleep aids. I'll give her your email address if you don't mind….

Jim

To: mGreenza@nhl.org
From: mGreenwood@powersleep.org
RE: Sleep Aids

Hi Mike!

Congratulations on getting to the semi-finals! Dr. Maas asked me to lend some advice about the use of sleep aids in stressful situations. As a clinical psychologist who sees a lot of patients with sleep disorders, I get this question all the time. Whether it's a business executive working on a big project or a family member dealing with the loss of a loved one, I usually tell them that over-the-counter (OTC) sleep aids are a safe and effective way of getting through stressful times as long as their doctors approve and they're careful not to become dependent on them. However, their use by athletes has some *special* considerations. Let me give you a quick overview of the most popular OTC medications, as well as some additional info about natural sleep remedies and prescription drugs:

OTC Meds
WARNING: with all meds in the sports world, athletes have to pay strict attention to banned substances. According to the USADA, there are many meds on the market that contain "pseudoephedrine or ephedrine derivatives and are therefore prohibited in competition. Often, but not always, these products have "D" in the name, for example Claritin-D and Benadryl-D."

Benadryl is an antihistamine used to treat sneezing, runny nose, and allergies. But because it promotes drowsiness, it is also commonly used as a sleep aid, taken about 30 minutes before bed. Side effects may include dizziness, headaches and temporary confusion, all of which can negatively impact athletic performance, especially if taken the night before a big game.

Nytol is another antihistamine, but it's used primarily as a sedative. It can also cause dizziness, and the label warns of potential fainting if used while exerting yourself in warm temperatures. Since it can get pretty hot in some arenas, this might not be your best choice. Most importantly, antihistamines block histamine receptors thus weakening the natural "thirst" response. When that thirst response is blocked, you may forget to drink that extra water bottle and you may notice that "dry mouth" sensation which is certainly a clue that you are dehydrated.

Tylenol PM is largely for easing those aches and pains that prevent you from falling and staying asleep. Its active ingredient (acetaminophen) does the physical soothing while a partner medicine (Simply Sleep) acts as a sedative. Side effects include dizziness, confusion, headache and dry mouth. The positive side of using meds that contain acetaminophen is that they will also help soothe aches and pains from practice the day before.

Overview
In review, OTC sleeping aids can help you fall asleep and perhaps stay asleep longer, but they should not be the only solution.

Yes, you may feel temporary relief in your ability to fall asleep quickly, but some of these aids actually inhibit your "deep sleep" which is crucial to your game. Due to the side effects, particularly next day drowsiness, I would not recommend experimenting with the sleep aids the very night before the game. A week or so before the big day

you can begin to work on figuring out which aide is best for you and your sleep habits.

Be sure to check the banned substances since some OTC medications may be prohibited. Remember, these remedies should not be used long term (to avoid dehydration, addiction etc). If you continue to have sleep problems, turn to your doctor to try and find a different solution.

Natural Remedies
Melatonin is a natural hormone produced by the pineal gland. It's nicknamed the "Hormone of Darkness" because its level increases as the sun sets, promoting sleep, and then decreases as morning arrives, promoting wakefulness. Some studies have found that taking melatonin supplements can induce sleep, and there are few if any immediate side effects. However, in the U.S., melatonin is not regulated by the FDA. So you can't be sure of its purity or even that a pill contains any melatonin at all. In fact, it is banned in the UK and Canada since they consider the medication a "drug" and have been held up in political and financial disputes due to the public's tendency to become addicted. In the United States, however, melatonin is considered a "supplement" allowing for the medication to be readily available to the public.

Valerian Root is a plant that is said to reduce the amount of time it takes to fall asleep. Some side effects include a "hangover" feeling, excitability, heart disturbances, and morning grogginess. Although this natural remedy may have a less intense sensation of drowsiness, it is still effective in relaxing a stressed athlete and helping promote sleep.

L-Tryptophan is another relative close to melatonin that can be used as a natural sleep aid. Do you ever wonder why you are so tired after Thanksgiving dinner? Perhaps it's due to the fact that turkey is a key source of L-Tryptophan, which is a hormone that has shown to help improve the sleep you get. You certainly don't have to run to the pharmacy to get that "sleepy" feeling on Thanksgiving Day.

Overview
Natural remedies are more readily available to the public and are slightly less risky for athletes. Many of them show similar side effects to the OTC sleep aides, but researchers argue they are safer and have fewer side effects.

The natural remedies may be a better option for athletes to help calm the pregame sleep jitters and anxiety. I would suggest, like the OTC medications, that you don't wait until the night before the game to experiment. I would also recommend that you and your doctor discuss the interactions of the sleep aids with any other medications you may be taking.

Prescription Drugs
*Quick key things to know about prescription sleep medications for athletes.

You should consult with a doctor about the prescribed sleeping medications because they are particularly more likely to cause addictions and abuse. Some countries, such as Australia, also ban the sleeping aides in fear that they might cause a vicious cycle of addiction in the athletes.

These medications should only be used for a short

period of time during stressful life events (training or games) because of possible rebound insomnia, in which people's mental dependency on the meds causes them to worry even more about not being able to fall asleep when they are no longer taking the pills. Furthermore, most sleeping pills keep you in deep sleep while reducing time in REM sleep. When you stop taking the medication there is a chance that you will experience a REM rebound effect. You'll spend more time in REM sleep to make up for the loss, and this will often include highly emotional and disturbing nightmares.

Like all other sleeping aides, I do not recommend that you take your first Ambien the night before the playoffs. Like all drugs, people have different reactions to the medicine. Although certain drugs claim that there will be no next-day drowsiness or headaches, you never know how your body will react and you certainly don't want to take that chance on game day!

Ambien is a time-released, two-layered non-benzodiazepine sedative-hypnotic drug that claims to "help you fall asleep fast and stay asleep." Side effects include headaches, dizziness, and a type of "amnesia" where you may not remember sleep walking or eating several hours after taking the pill.

Ambien may have an increased risk of tolerance just like any drug in that your body gets accustomed to the drug and you have to increase dosage. The risk of dependence on Ambien for the ability to fall asleep (rebound insomnia when not taking the pill), withdrawal, and unusual changes in behavior such as confusion, aggression, agitation, hallucinations and suicidal thoughts are high in Ambien users.

Once discussed with your doctor, the use of Ambien on a short-term basis may be effective for athletes, particularly in relation to jet lag. The drug doesn't tend to produce the same next day drowsiness that the OTC medications do which may make or break your performance.

Lunesta is a non-narcotic drug that is also supposed to help you fall asleep and stay asleep, but has a lower risk of tolerance when used over time and of encountering "rebound insomnia." However, side effects still include drowsiness, dizziness, dependence, headache, and congestion. There have also been reports of memory loss, anxiety, allergic reactions, and abnormal thoughts. Lunesta is similar to Ambien in helping athletes sleep through stressful weeks of training or games but it is considered a less habit-forming drug.

Rozerem is said to be the first sleep drug to have little-to-no risk of dependence or abuse. It selectively targets receptors in the brain that control your internal biological clock. Common side effects include dizziness, headache, stuffy nose, nausea, diarrhea, and a sore throat. Lunesta and Rozerem are popular among athlete forums. Many consider the two as the better option than Ambien because they are simply less dangerous, addictive and performance affecting.

Overview
As you can see, prescription sleep aids carry significant risk. In your case, the extra rest they provide may be counteracted by the side effects they produce. I generally only recommend them to patients suffering chronic insomnia after natural remedies and OTC meds have failed to help. And even then, they should only be used temporarily

and selectively so as not to develop a dependence on them.

People who wouldn't ordinarily take prescription sleep aids sometimes pop one on a long plane flight to insure they get enough rest. But in your case, I would not recommend that because the drugs are risky and you need to be prepared to dedicate at least eight hours of solid sleep.

Lastly, some research has suggested that prescription medications, such as Ambien, may promote longer time spent in deep sleep. Researchers make the argument that deeper sleep promotes muscle repair and recovery which may help you to wake up feeling refreshed and ready to play!

With that said, I would still suggest trying out the natural and OTC medications before turning to prescription medications. Don't experiment with any of the above within days of the games. Just like practice, its crucial to try out the different medications before settling on one. Make sure this happens well in advance with the help of a doctor and your trainer. Remember to cross reference the list of approved medications so that you and your teammates don't get in trouble with the league!

That's my best advice, Mike. If you have any questions, let me know. Otherwise, good luck!

Maura Greenwood

12 A Fairytale Ending?

In the weeks that followed, the Flyers slipped past the Bruins in seven and then faced off against the New York Islanders for the Stanley Cup. I watched every second of every game from my living room in Ithaca, cheering for each Philadelphia goal and pounding the couch in frustration after every questionable call. My wife even bought me a Flyers' jersey – No. 19, of course – which I proudly wore through it all. You would have thought one of my own sons was out there on the ice; that's how big a fan I became.

Mike continued to play like a star. He had the assist on the series-winning goal against Boston and then scored four goals in the first five games of the finals, leading his team to a 3-2 series lead. I had the champagne iced in my living room for the sixth game in New York, but the Islanders scored twice in the final period to send the series back to Philadelphia for the seventh and deciding game.

The next afternoon I got an email from Mike, inviting my wife and me to Philly for the final game the following night. I actually had to read it twice because I couldn't believe he'd extended such an invitation. "Two seats, center ice, right behind the Flyers bench...because whatever happens, you helped bring us here and you deserve to be a part of it."

We drove through New York and down the Pennsylvania Turnpike on a gloomy, early-spring morning. But the weather was of no consequence to me. Over the years advising athletic teams, I'd been blessed with many great experiences, but this, regardless of how it turned out, was probably the most exciting one of all.

That evening, Broad Street and the Wells Fargo Center was a mob scene. Traffic was so thick, we just managed to get to our seats as the house lights went down and the national anthem was being sung. I actually had goosebumps under my Flyers jersey.

Mike somehow found us in the crowd and gave me a smile and a thumbs-up sign before skating out to center ice. In the midst of it all, he looked remarkably confident, calm and, if I do say so myself, well-rested.

But the Flyers struggled through the first two periods, stymied by a tenacious Islander defense that held them to just a dozen shots on goal. Fortunately, New York's offense wasn't much better. At the beginning of the third period, it was Islanders 1, Flyers 0.

Now I am not what you'd call a fervently religious man, but as the clock ticked down I started praying. Everyone was on their feet, the collective roar of the crowd rising in anticipation with each Flyer breakaway and then falling in disappointment every time it was thwarted.

But then, with four minutes left to go, an Islander defenseman was called for hooking, and on the ensuing power play Mike tucked in a rebound for the tying goal.

I not only hugged my wife, but I also hugged the guy next to me, the guy in front of me, and quite possibly one of the ushers. I don't remember, I was so excited! Once things settled down, the Flyers expertly killed off what remained of regulation and, unbelievably, we were heading for overtime.

Given how I felt in the stands, I couldn't imagine how Mike and his teammates were keeping it together on the ice. Remarkably, Coach Harkwell didn't give them any special pep talk in between periods. I watched as he simply walked down the bench and gave each one a pat on the shoulder. I guess when you get to a point like this, no special words or plays will get you any further. It's just a matter of how much you want it.

The Flyers didn't wait long. Riding the momentum of their

game-tying goal, they came out skating with a coordinated ferocity like none I've ever witnessed. They peppered the Islander goalie with shot after shot as the whole stadium roared and rocked until...until things suddenly went into slow motion for me and, I'm sure, for Mike as well.

A Flyer defenseman stole the puck and hit Mike on a breakaway up the left wing. He deked one Islander, then another, and – everyone knew what would happen next – slid toward the crease and – at 13:54 of overtime – flicked the puck over the goalie's right shoulder.

The place exploded.

I remember cheering and crying at the same time, while out on the ice Mike and his teammates paraded and kissed the Stanley Cup with tears on their cheeks as well. In time, the PA announcer broke in to say Mike had been voted the series MVP.

Somehow in this throng Mike managed to find me. He pumped my hand, gave me a hug, then grabbed my arm and skated me toward the far side of the arena. In a daze, I exited the ice and stumbled up a walkway, down a concrete corridor, and into the Flyers' locker room. It was just as loud in here as it was out there.

"Hey! Hey!" Mike screamed as he pulled me up on a makeshift platform used for TV interviews. "I want to introduce you to someone! This is Professor Maas, the sleep coach!"

And with that I was drenched by a shower of champagne and an actual cheer went up. I have to admit, in that moment I felt like I had scored the winning goal in overtime in the seventh and deciding game of the Stanley Cup finals.

And then, and then....

I felt someone shaking me as the scene began to fade....

"Jim! Jim!"

The voice of my worried wife.

"Are you all right? Wake up!"

And I slowly, stubbornly, returned to reality, to my bedroom in Ithaca, to the thoughts of the classes I had to teach today....

Had it really all been a dream?

But then, as I rolled over onto my side, trying to return to wherever I'd been for just one minute more, I felt something in my pajama pocket.

It was – could it really be? – a champagne cork: Moet Chandon 1993.

Appendices

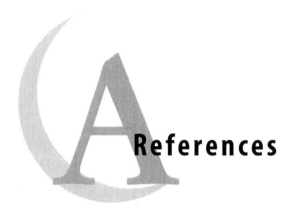

References

Chapter 5

1. Mah CD; Mah KE; Kezirian EJ; Dement WC. The effects of sleep extension on the athletic performance of collegiate basketball players. SLEEP 2011; 34(7): 943-950.

2. Potenziano BJ et al. Sleepiness as a predictor of player longevity within major league baseball. SLEEP 2012; 35, Abs 0810:A273.

3. Rogers SL et al. Sleepiness as a predictor of draft value in the National Football League. SLEEP 2012; 35, Abs 0211:A76.

4. Winter WC, M.D., medical director, Martha Jefferson Hospital Sleep Medicine Center at Charlottesville, Va.; Carl Boethel, M.D., medical director, Scott & White Sleep Institute, Temple, Texas; June 9, 2010, presentation, SLEEP 2010, San Antonio.

5. Smith RS et al. Circadian Rhythms and Enhanced Athletic Performance in the National Football League. Sleep, 20(5): 362-365.

6. Budgett R. Fatigue and underperformance in athletes: the overtraining syndrome. Br J Sports Med 1998; 32: 107-110.

7. Van Cauter E and Leproult R. Role of Sleep and Sleep Loss in Hormonal Release and Metabolism. Endocr Dev; 17; 11-21.

8. Shapiro CM, Bortz R, Mitchell D, Bartel P, Jooste P. Slow-wave sleep: a recovery period after exercise. Science. 1981 Dec 11; 214(4526): 1253-4.

Chapter 7

1. Forbes-Robertson S, et al. Circadian Disruption and Remedial Interventions. Sports Med 2012; 42(3): 185-208.
2. Waterhouse J, Reilly T, Atkinson G, Edwards B. Jet lag: trends and coping strategies. The Lancet. 2007 March 31; Vol 369: 1117-9.

Chapter 8

1. Litvin, E.B., Ditre, J.W., Heckman, B.W., & Brandon, T. H. (2012). Nicotine. *Drug Abuse and Addiction in Medical Illness*, 137-150.
2. Tassinari, C. A., Ambrosetto, G., Peraita-Adrados, M. R., & Gastaut, H. (1976). The neuropsychiatric syndrome of delta-9-tetrahydrocannabinol and cannabis intoxication in naive subjects: A clinical and polygraphic study during wakefulness and sleep. *Pharmacology of Marijuana*, 357-375.
3. Freemon, F.R. (1972). Effects of marijuana on sleeping states. *JAMA, 220,* 1364-1365.
4. Kales, A., Hanley, J., Rickles, W., Kanas, N., Baker, M., & Goring, P. (1972). Effects of marijuana administration and withdrawal in chronic users and naive subjects. *Psychophysiology, 9,* 92.
5. Halikas, J.A., Weller, R.A., Morse, C.L., & Hoffman, R.G. (1985). A longitudinal study of marijuana effects. *The International Journal of the Addictions, 20,* 701-711.
6. Bolla, K.I., Lesage, S.R., Gamaldo, C.E., Neubauer, D.N., Funderburk, F.R., Cadet, J.L., David, P.M., Verdeio-Garcia, A. & Benbrook, A.R. (2008). Sleep disturbance in heavy marijuana users. *Sleep, 31,* 901-908.
7. Nicholson, A. N., Turner, C., Stone, B. M., & Robson, P.

J. (2004). Effect of [DELTA]-9-tetrahydrocannabinol and cannabidiol on nocturnal sleep and early-morning behavior in young adults. *Journal of Clinical Psychopharmacology, 24,* 305-313.

8. Schneiker, K.T., Bishop, D., Dawson, B., & Hackett, L.P. (2006). Effects of caffeine on prolonged intermittent-sprint ability in team-sport athletes. *Medicine and Science in Sport and Exercise, 38,* 578-585.

9. Smit, H.J., & Rogers, P.J. (2000). Effects of low doses of caffeine on cognitive performance, mood and thirst in low and higher caffeine consumers. *Psychopharmacology, 152,* 167-173.

10. Volpe, S.L. (2010). Alcohol and Athletic Performance. *ACSM's Health & Fitness Journal, 14,* 28-30.

11. Gutgesell, M., & Canterbury R. (1999). Alcohol usage in sport and exercise. *Addiction Biology, 4,* 373-383.

12. Boone T, Gilmore S. Effects of sexual intercourse on maximal aerobic power, oxygen pulse, and double product in male sedentary subjects (1995). *Journal of Sports Medicine and Physical Fitness , 35,* 214-217.

13. Hamilton LD, & Meston C. (2010). The role of salivary cortisol and DHEA-S in response to sexual, humorous, and anxiety-inducing stimuli. *Hormones and Behavior,* Dec 30.

14. Hamilton L.D., Rellini A., & Meston C. (2008) Cortisol, sexual arousal, and affect in response to sexual stimuli. *Journal of Sexual Medicine, 5,* 2111-2118.

15. Dabbs J, Mohammed S. (1992) Male and female salivary testosterone concentrations before and after sexual activity. *Physiology & Behaviour* 52:1, 195-197

16. Komisaruk, B.R., & Whipple, B. (1995). The suppression of pain by genital stimulation in females. *Annual Review of Sex Research, 6,* 151-186.

17. Jowett, S., & Cramer, D. (2009). The role of romantic

relationships on athletes' performance and well-being. *Journal of Clinical Sport Psychology, 3,* 58-72.

Additional:

1. Barratt, E.S., Beaver, W. & White, R. (1974). The effects of marijuana on human sleep patterns. *Biological Psychiatry, 8,* 47-54.

2. Feinberg, I., Jones, R., Walker, J.M., Cavness, C., & March, J. (1975). Effects of high dosage delta-9-tetrahydrocannabinol on sleep patterns in man. *Clinical Pharmacology & Therapeutics, 17,* 458-466.

3. Feinberg, I., Jones, R., Walker, J., Cavness, C., & Floyd, T. (1976). Effects of marijuana extract and tetrahydrocannabinol on electroencephalographic sleep patterns. *Clinical pharmacology and therapeutics, 19,* 782.-794.

Chapter 9

1. Coggan AR, Coyle EF. *Carbohydrate Ingestion During Prolonged Exercise: Effects on Metabolism and Performance.* Exerc Sport Sci Rev. 1991;19:1-40.

2. Coyle, EF, et al. *Carbohydrate Feeding During Prolonged Strenuous Exercise Can Delay Fatigue.* J Appl Physiol. 1983 Jul;55(1 Pt 1):230-5.

3. Currell K, Jeukendrup AE. *Superior Endurance Performance With Ingestion of Multiple Transportable Carbohydrates.* Med Sci Sports Exerc, 2008;40:275–81.

4. Hawley JA, et al. *Promoting Training Adaptations Through Nutritional Interventions.* J. Sports Sci, 24(7):709-721.

5. Jentjens RLPG., Achten, J., Jeukendrup AE. High oxidation rates from combined carbphydrates ingested during exercise. Med Sci Sports Exerc 2004: 36 (9): 1551-1558.

6. Jentjens RLPG., Underwood K., Achten, J., Currell K., Mann CH, Asker E., Jeukendrup AE. Exogenous carbohydrate oxidation rates are elevated after combined ingestion of glucose

and fructose during exercise in the heat. J Appl Physiol 2006; 100: 807-816.

7. Jeukendrup A. *Carbohydrate Supplementation During Exercise: Does it Help? How Much is Too Much?* Gatorade Sports Sci Exch. 2007;20:1–5. Gatorade Sports Science Institute Web site [Internet]. 2007.

8. Lunn, WR, Pasiakos, SM, et. Al. *Chocolate Milk and Endurance Exercise Recovery: Protein Balance, Glycogen, and Performance.* Medicine & Science in Sports & Exercise, April 2012 - Volume 44 - Issue 4 - p 682–691.

9. Martínez-Lagunas V, Ding Z, Bernard JR, Wang B, Ivy JL. *Added Protein Maintains Efficacy of a Low-Carbohydrate Sports Drink.* J Strength Cond Res, 2010 Jan;24(1):48-59.

10. McConell G, et al. *Effect of Timing of Carbohydrate Ingestion on Endurance Exercise Performance.* Med Sci Sports Exerc. 1996;28:1300-4.

11. Millard-Stafford ML, et al. *Carbohydrate-Electrolyte Replacement Improves Distance Running Performance in the Heat.* Med Sci Sports Exerc. 1992 Aug;24(8):934-40

12. Nicholas CW, et al. *Influence of Ingesting a Carbohydrate-Electrolyte Solution on Endurance Capacity During Intermittent, High-Intensity Shuttle Running.* J Sports Sci. 1995 Aug;13(4):283-90.

13. Van Essen MJ, Gibala, MJ. *Failure of Protein to Improve Time Trial Performance When Added To a Sports Drink.* Med Sci Sports Exerc. 38:1476-1483, 2006.

14. Wilber RL and Moffatt RJ. *Physiological and Biomechanical Consequences of Detraining in Aerobically Trained Individuals.* Journal of Strength Conditioning Research, 8:110.

Chapter 10

1. Pesca M. Sports injuries: A look at the data. National Public Radio. 2012 May 20. [Audio podcast].

2. Shapiro CM, Bortz R, Mitchell D, Bartel P, Jooste P. Slow-

eave sleep: a recovery period after exercise. Science. 1981 Dec 11; 214(4526): 1253-4.

Chapter 11

1. Eidi M, Oryan S, Eidi A, Sepehrara L. Effect of morphine, naloxone and histamine system on water intake in adult male rats. Eur J Pharmacol. 2003;478(2-3):105-10.
2. "Examples of Prohibited Substances & Methods." USADA, 1 2011. Web. 23 Dec 2012. <http://www.usada.org/files/active/ athletes/wallet_card.pdf>.
3. Maas JB & Robbins RS. "Sleep for Success! Everything You Must Know About Sleep But Are Too Tired to Ask: 9781452037752: (204-214). N.p., n.d. Web. 23 Dec. 2012.

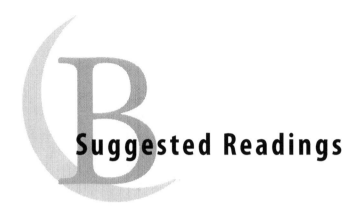

Suggested Readings

Carskadon, Mary A. *The Encyclopedia of Sleep and Dreaming.* New York: MacMillan, 1993.

Dement, William C. *The Promise of Sleep.* New York: Random House, 1999

Dinges, David and Roger Broughton. *Sleep and Alertness: Chronological, Behavioral and Medical Aspects of Napping.* New York: Raven, 1990.

Epstein, L. *Improving Sleep.* Cambridge MA: Harvard Health Publications, 2010.

Kryger, Meir. *A Good Night's Sleep.* New York: Metro Books, 2009.

Maas, James B. "Who Needs Sleep?" Ithaca, NY: Cornell University, 2006 (DVD for teens. Available from www.jamesmaas.com)

Maas, James B. *Power Sleep. Hardcover.* New York: Random House, 1998.

Maas. James B. *Power Sleep.* Paperback ed. New York: Harper Collions, 1999.

Maas, James B., Robbins, Rebecca S, *Sleep for Success.* Bloomington, IN: AuthorHouse, 2011.

Maas, James B. *Remmy and the Brain Train. Ithaca, NY: Maas Publications, 2001.*

Maas, James B., Robbins, Rebecca S., et.al. *Encyclopedia of Adolescence*, chapter on "Adolescent Sleep." Oxford, UK: Elsevier, 2011,

Mednick, Sara C. Take a Nap! Change Your Life. New York: Workman Publishing Co., 2006

Reite, Martin, Ruddy, J, and Nagel, Kim. *Evaluation and Management of Sleep Disorders*, 3rd ed. Washington, D.C.: American Psychiatric Publishing, Inc. 2002.

Schneck, Carlos. Sleep: The Mysteries, The Problems, and The Solutions. New York: Avery, 2007.

Sleep to Win, LLC.

Life changing keynote presentations, training programs and seminars

Almost everybody is sleep deprived. To be a peak performer you need to be fully alert, dynamic, energetic, in a good mood, and cognitively sharp. This is possible only through quality sleep.

Our multi-media presentations, extremely popular with corporations, educational institutions, athletic franchises and general audiences, focus on giving you the tools to radically jumpstart your life. We will answer questions such as:

- What are the consequences of sleep deprivation on thinking, performance, health, and lifespan?
- What are the four golden rules and ten sleep strategies that will assure you a great night's sleep and a better tomorrow?
- What are the five stages of nocturnal sleep, and why are they essential for maximum functioning?
- How can you reduce travel fatigue?
- How can you increase your athletic performance overnight?
- Do you need less sleep as you get older?
- Can you learn while you sleep?
- Can napping improve cognitive abilities?
- How do you choose a great pillow and mattress?
- What causes insomnia, and how can it be overcome?

The information provided will increase your daytime alertness, psychological mood, productivity, creativity, and quality of life. Our programs will show you highly specific behaviors and routines that will enhance your life immediately. The Sleep for Success training module can be delivered in a variety of ways, and customized to fit your organization's specific needs.

Dr. James B. Maas is one of the world's most noted award-winning teachers. He taught more than 65,000 university students in his 48 years on the Cornell University faculty, where he served as professor and chair of Psychology and was a Weiss Presidential Fellow. He is the recipient of the American Psychological Association's Distinguished Educator Award, was a visiting professor at Stanford University and a Fulbright Senior Lecturer to Sweden. Sleep to Win Vice President Haley Davis is an expert in sleep research and education and the author of several articles on sleep and well-being.

The staff of Sleep to Win have presented highly successful programs on sleep to scores of corporations, athletes, athletic franchises, educational institutions and medical audiences. Clients include IBM, GAP, Google, Goldman Sachs, CitiGroup, JP Morgan Chase, Starwood Hotels, Crystal Cruise Lines, the American College of Facial and Plastic Surgeons, the American College of Rheumatology, the American Urological Association, Campbell's Soups, Pepsi Cola, the US Navy, the United States Figure Skating

Association, the New York Jets, the Philadelphia Flyers, the Ottawa Senators, the Orlando Magic, and the Young President's Organization.

For more information on Sleep to Win! keynote presentations, seminars and workshops, contact Dr. James B. Maas at maas.james@gmail.com and visit www.sleeptowin.com.

To order Dr. Maas pillows, bedding products, and other sleeping aids designed to promote better sleep, go to:

www.bedbathandbeyond.com (Dr. Maas Pillows)
www.paramountsleep.com (Dr. Maas Collection)
www.myzeo.com
www.litebook.com

About the Authors

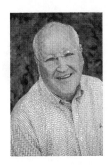

Dr. James B. Maas is a leading authority and international consultant on sleep and performance who has studied the subject more than four decades. Dr. Maas received his BA from Williams College and his MA and PhD from Cornell and was a Weiss Presidential Fellow, professor and former chair of Cornell University's psychology department. The author of *Power Sleep*, he lives in Fort Worth, Texas.

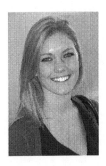

Haley A. Davis is vice-president of the Sleep to Win consulting firm. She is completing her BS in psychology and pre-med at Cornell University, where she has been conducting research and publishing articles on sleep.

87758577R00081

Made in the USA
Columbia, SC
18 January 2018